Patients Beyond Borders™
Turkey Edition

Everybody's Guide to Affordable,
World-Class Medical Tourism

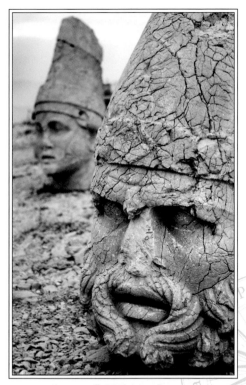

Josef Woodman

HEALTHY TRAVEL MEDIA

www.patientsbeyondborders.com

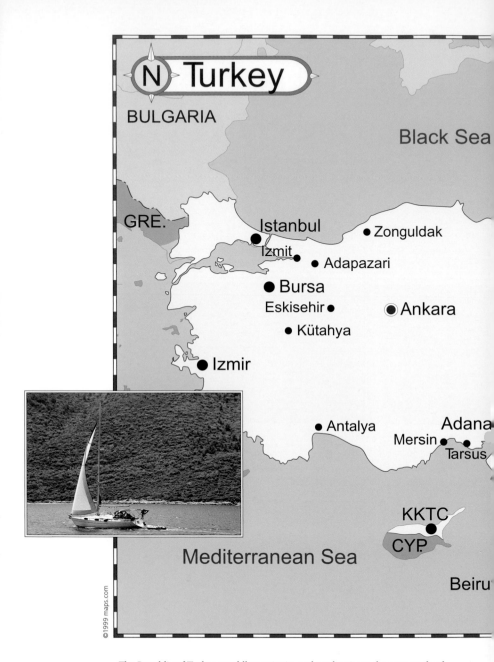

The Republic of Turkey straddles antiquity and modernity at the crossroads of Europe, Asia, and the Middle East. It shares borders with eight other countries, and its coastline runs along three seas. Asian Turkey, made up largely of the Anatolian Peninsula, is 97 percent of the country. The remainder, eastern Thrace or Rumelia in the Balkan Peninsula, is European Turkey. The two are separated by the Sea of Marmara and the Istanbul and Dardanelles Bosphorus, which together form a water link between the Black Sea and the Mediterranean.

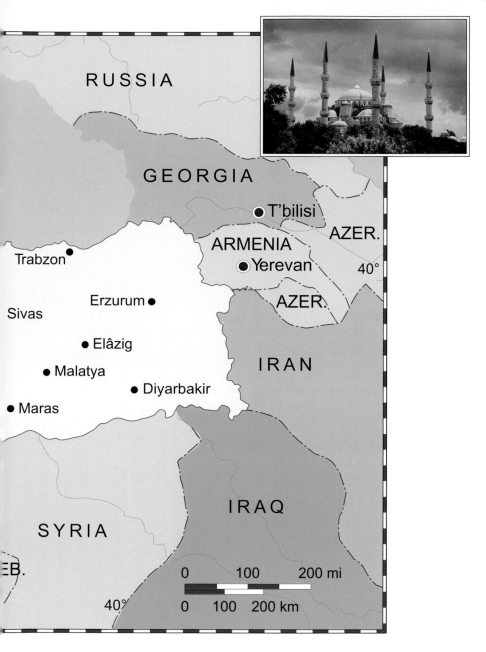

Rising from west to east, the country's elevation reaches about 2,600 feet (800 meters) above sea level in central Anatolia and 7,200 feet (2,200 meters) in eastern Anatolia—home to Turkey's highest peak, Mount Ararat, or Everest. Western Anatolia is a region of eroded mountain ranges, fertile valleys, meandering rivers, peninsulas, and bays. Most medical travelers to this uniquely Eurasian nation seek services in one of its three prominent "cities of health": Istanbul and Izmir on the coast, and Turkey's capital, Ankara, in central Anatolia.

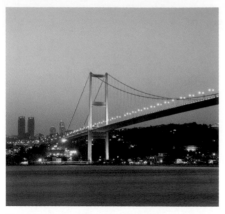

The Bosphorus Bridge, Istanbul

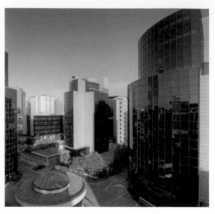

The Maslak financial region

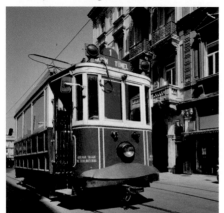

Tram in Istiklal Caddesi, Taksim

Istanbul, where the hearts of two continents beat with history, culture, art, and music.

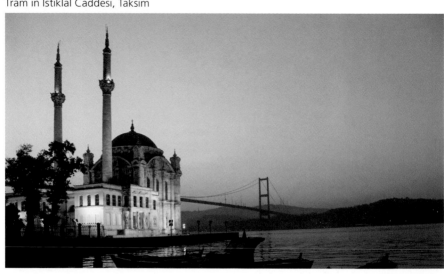

Evening serenity at the Ortakoy Mosque

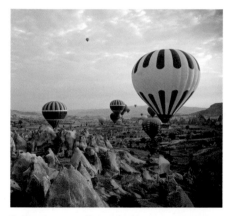

Ballooning over Cappadocia

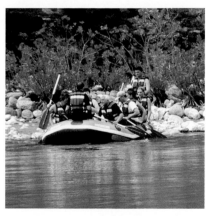

Rafting the Coruh River

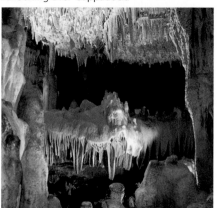

Damlatas Cave, Antalya

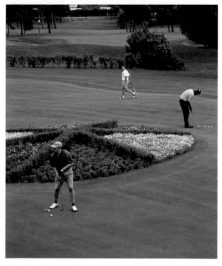

World-class golf courses

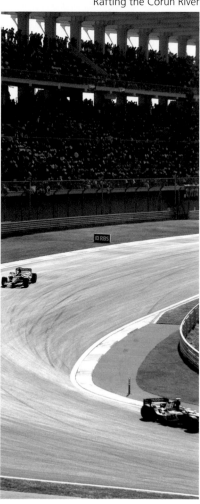

Formula 1 races in Istanbul

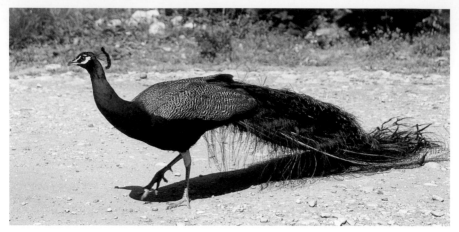

Proud peacock

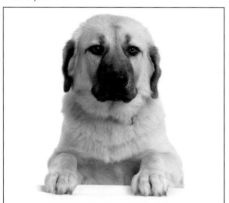

Turkey offers
a multitude of
indigenous
species and
cultures.

Sivas Kangal watchdog

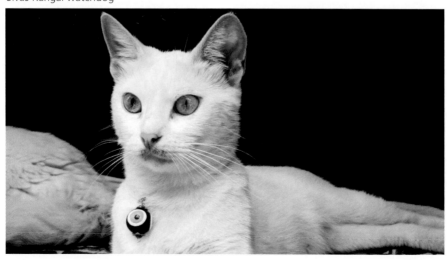

Van cat, another unique Turkish breed

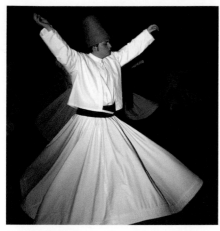

Ritual of the Whirling Dervishes

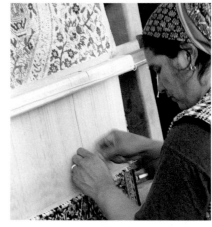

Handlooming in Alanya

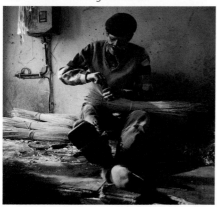

Traditional broom craftsman

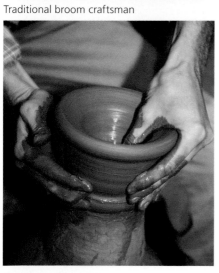

Classical Turkish pottery

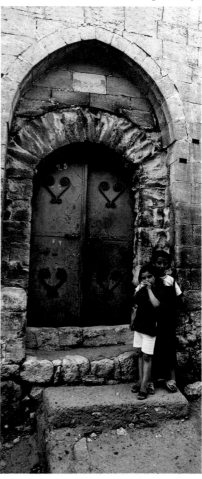

Old house in Diyarbakir

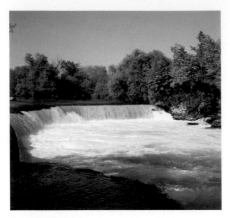

Koprulu Canyon

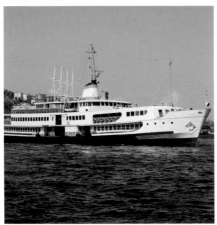

Ferrying to the other side of Istanbul

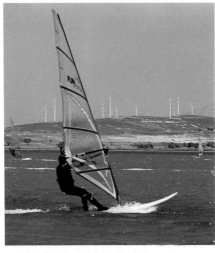

Windsurfing in Cesme, Alacati

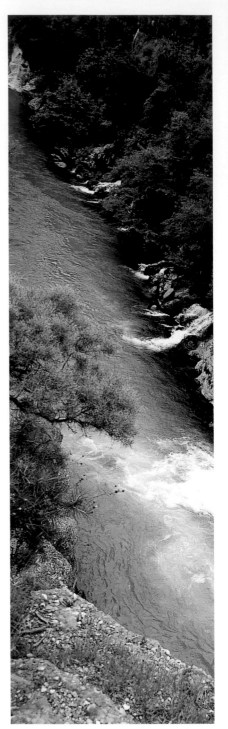

The historical Euphrates River

"A useful new book on this topic . . ."

—*Savvy Senior*

"I am considering elective surgery and this was a great compendium of information scattered all over the Internet."

—Amy Tupper (Sanford, NC)

"I spent a lot of time on the Internet trying to research this topic on my own and looking for certain procedures (mainly dental and cosmetic surgery). I wound up getting dental work done in Mexico at a facility reviewed in [*Patients Beyond Borders*] and am happy with my experience. I recommend this book to anyone even remotely considering foreign medical travel."

— K. Williamson (Los Lunas, NM)

"If the American healthcare system is not completely broken, it is certainly dysfunctional: 47 million people have no health coverage, and 130 million have no dental insurance. As baby boomers age into more medical problems with spotty coverage and would prefer not to deplete their retirement savings, they are looking at all available options."

—*Financial Times*

"A must-read for those considering medical tourism . . ."

—*ABC News*

"A practical guide to planning a medical trip . . ."

—*Washington Post*

Patients Beyond Borders Series™

Patients Beyond Borders™
Turkey Edition

Everybody's Guide to Affordable,
World-Class Medical Tourism

Josef Woodman

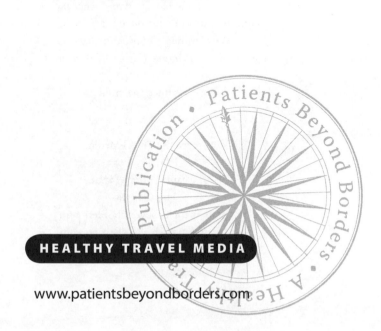

HEALTHY TRAVEL MEDIA

www.patientsbeyondborders.com

PATIENTS BEYOND BORDERS: TURKEY EDITION
Everybody's Guide to Affordable, World-Class Medical Tourism

Copyright © 2009 by Josef Woodman

ISBN 13: 978-0-9823361-1-3

Cover Art and Page Design: Anne Winslow
Developmental Editing: Faith Brynie
Copyediting: Kate Johnson
Proofreading: Barbara Resch
Indexing: Madge Walls
Color Layout: Judy Orchard
Typesetting and Production: Copperline Book Services
POD Printing: Catawba Publishing, LLC
Offset Printing: C & C Offset Printers

Printed in China

Healthy Travel Media
P.O. Box 17057
Chapel Hill, NC 27516
919 370.7380
info@patientsbeyondborders.com
www.patientsbeyondborders.com

To All the Dedicated Healthcare Workers of Turkey

Limits of Liability and Disclaimer of Warranty
Please Read Carefully

This book is intended as a reference guide, not as a medical guide or manual for self-diagnosis or self-treatment. While the intent of *Patients Beyond Borders: Turkey Edition* is to provide useful and informative data, neither the author nor any other party affiliated with this book renders or recommends the use of specific hospitals, clinics, professional services (including physicians and surgeons), third-party agencies, or any other source cited throughout this book.

Patients Beyond Borders: Turkey Edition should not be used as a substitute for advice from a medical professional. The author and publisher expressly disclaim responsibility for any adverse effects that might arise from the information found in *Patients Beyond Borders: Turkey Edition* or any other book, Web site, or information associated with *Patients Beyond Borders*. Readers who suspect they may have a specific medical problem should consult a physician about any suggestions made in this book.

Hospitals, clinics, or any other treatment institution cited throughout *Patients Beyond Borders: Turkey Edition* are responsible for all treatment provided to patients, including but not limited to surgical, medical, wellness, beauty, and all related queries, opinions, and complications. The author, publisher, editors, and all other parties affiliated with this book are not responsible for same, including any emergency, complication, or medical requirement of whatsoever nature, arising from the patient's treatment due to the patient's present or past illness, or the side effects of drugs or lack of adequate treatment. All pre-treatments, treatments, and post-treatments are the absolute responsibility of the hospital, clinic, or any other treating institution, and/or the treating physician.

ACKNOWLEDGMENTS

"At first my publisher had reservations about publishing it in the form you are familiar with."
—Orhan Pamuk, *Turkish Novelist, Nobel Laureate*

EVERY WORTHWHILE PUBLISHED work is a group effort; any author who tells you differently is lying or hopelessly grandiose! *Patients Beyond Borders: Turkey Edition* is certainly no exception, and is the collective result of so many able and talented individuals. The people I met during these months of research and production have rewarded me with the unique richness of Turkish hospitality, humor, and a collaborative spirit so vital to a successful publishing outcome.

My deepest thanks go out to Meri Bahar of the Accredited Hospitals Association of Turkey, for her early vision on this project. I shall not soon forget her very-early-morning impromptu telephone call ("We wish you to publish a book, how soon may we see it in print?"), beginning a rewarding 18-month journey that led to the work you now hold in your hands. Meri worked relentlessly with their newly formed association to help fund this project and bring it to life.

Faith Brynie and David Boucher provided initial encouragement in having me seriously examine Turkey as a medical travel destination. I am grateful to Dr. Sina Ercan, Tulpar Demirbilek,

Beril Ongen of the Healthcare Tourism Committee, Asli Akyavas, and Hasan Kus for their early support and editorial contributions. And a special note of appreciation goes to Melis Zorluoglu, who spent far more of her life these past few months than she might ever have imagined, attending to the endless details of keeping the project on track, and bringing all the details to fruition. Thanks also to Prof. Dr. Sevil Kutay, president of the Turkish American Chamber of Commerce and Industry Midwest.

Finally, a heartfelt note of appreciation to the editors, proofreaders, designers, and indexer who made the Turkey Edition possible. Special thanks to Faith Brynie, who crafted the manuscript; to Kate Johnson, who managed the editorial process in sometimes choppy waters; and to Judy Orchard and Nicki Florence, for their meticulous attention to detail on the color pages.

Josef Woodman
Chapel Hill, NC
2009

Contents

PART TWO: TURKEY: A PRIME DESTINATION FOR THE MEDICAL TRAVELER

PART THREE: TURKEY: A NATION TO SEE AND LOVE

PART FOUR: RESOURCES AND REFERENCES

PREFACE TO THE TURKEY EDITION

WHAT A DIFFERENCE five years can make! When I first began researching *Patients Beyond Borders,* Turkey frequently surfaced as an important healthcare destination, yet remained—much like the literary lore surrounding its largest city, Istanbul—enigmatic and inaccessible. Today, following nearly two decades of government and private investment in healthcare, the results are manifest and impressive. By nearly every measure, Turkey's growth in healthcare has kept pace with its counterparts to the East *and* West. Specialty centers and clinics are opening by the month, offering patients nearly every imaginable procedure at Western standards of excellence, and at significant cost savings over their European and North American counterparts.

From traditional cardiovascular and orthopedic treatments to cutting-edge genetics, neurosurgery, and oncology, Turkey offers medical travelers the comfort of state-of-the-art facilities, quality assurance in care, and a friendly tourism infrastructure. Recent affiliations with prestigious US medical centers, such as Harvard, Mayo, Johns Hopkins, and Memorial Sloan-Kettering, bring shared research and best practices to both sides of the pond and enrich the patient experience.

Now, among Turkey's international hospitals are 12 percent of the world's Joint Commission International (JCI)–accredited facilities—more than in any other country.

Thus, it's no surprise that Turkey is one of the fastest-growing medical travel destinations, and its ministries of health and tourism are pouring hundreds of millions of dollars into welcoming patients from all over the globe. Turkey expects to attract more than 1 million foreign patients to its shores by 2015.

Geographically central as it is, Turkey is certainly well poised for such growth. Middle Easterners disenfranchised from the US healthcare system are embracing nearby Turkey, which offers cultural familiarity with an increasingly Western flair. For patients in Western and Central European economies that are beginning to buckle under the strain of universal healthcare, Turkey is a relatively short hop to avoid the sometimes long waits for procedures in their own countries. And for those in neighboring Eastern Europe and the Middle East, where quality healthcare is often not as advanced or varied, Turkey offers important and nearby choices.

Turkey's three principal "Healthcare Cities"—Istanbul, Ankara, and Izmir—are all worthy tourist destinations in their own rights, with good-sized international airports serving each. From Istanbul's unforgettably rich setting along the Golden Horn (a mere walk across a bridge from Europe to Asia), to Ankara's Hattian civilization relics, to the enticing Aegean shoreline of Izmir, Turkey has much to offer the medical traveler seeking to explore the country pre-procedure, or to recover in a land that some 12 million tourists visit each year.

And of course, Turkey is well known as one of the world's first medical travel destinations—its healing waters attracted Greeks seeking better health more than two millennia ago. Dozens of the world's best modern-day spas and wellness resorts are now found in Turkey's cities and resorts. For those seeking alternative therapies, complementary and wellness strategies, or simply a pampered recuperation experience, Turkey has it all.

It's a joy to see the world of medical care so rapidly and successfully evolve in Turkey, offering medical travelers a choice of robust and affordable options in such a welcoming, gracious country.

Josef Woodman
November 2009

Patients Beyond Borders Series™

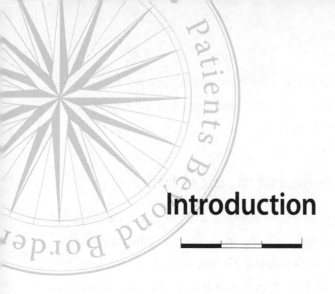

Introduction

If you're holding this copy of *Patients Beyond Borders: Turkey Edition* in your hands, you probably already know that you need a medical procedure, and perhaps you are considering an affordable, trustworthy alternative to care in your own country. As you can see, this is a specialty volume in the *Patients Beyond Borders* series, profiling the Republic of Turkey as a healthcare destination. It is intended for those who already have (more or less) a diagnosis and already know (more or less) what treatment they need.

This edition doesn't provide the breadth of general information about medical travel that you'll find in our larger book, *Patients Beyond Borders: Everybody's Guide to Affordable, World-Class Medical Travel*, now in its Second Edition. Instead, this volume first offers an overview of the questions you need to answer before you commit to medical travel; then, most of its pages are devoted to describing the best places in Turkey to find excellent treatment and care. It also contains information on health travel agents who can help you make the necessary arrangements in Turkey at a reasonable price.

The Phenomenon of Medical Travel

In the last three years, I have traveled to 22 countries and visited more than 140 hospitals, talking to surgeons, healthcare administrators, and their patients. Health travelers are often pleasantly surprised at the quality of care, the prices, and the all-around good experience of their medical travel abroad. As we contemplate our options in an overburdened healthcare environment, many of us will eventually find ourselves seeking alternatives to costly treatments—either for ourselves or for our loved ones. Healthcare consumers everywhere are in the midst of a global shift in medical services. In these few short years, big government investment, corporate partnerships, and increased media attention have spawned a new industry, medical tourism, bringing with it a host of encouraging new choices.

This new phenomenon of medical tourism—or international health travel—has recently received a good deal of wide-eyed attention. While one newspaper or blog giddily touts the fun 'n sun side of treatment abroad, another issues dire warnings about filthy hospitals, shady treatment practices, and procedures gone bad. As with most things in life, the truth lies somewhere in between. When I speak to interviewers and reporters, I try to emphasize that "medical tourism" is a misnomer. Medical travel is not a vacation. Unlike some other books on medical travel, this one focuses more on your health than on your recreational preferences. Business travelers don't consider themselves tourists; neither should you. This book will help you think about the "business" of health travel.

Patients Beyond Borders: Turkey Edition isn't a guide to medical diagnosis and treatment, nor does it provide medical advice on specific treatments or caregiver referrals. Your condition, diagnosis, treatment options, and travel preferences are unique, and only you—in consultation with your physician and loved ones—can determine the best course of action. Should you decide to go abroad for treatment, we provide a wealth of resources and tools to help you become an informed medical traveler, so you can have the best possible travel experience and treatment your money can buy.

My research, including countless interviews, has convinced me that with diligence, perseverance, and good information, patients considering traveling to Turkey or any other country for treatment indeed have legitimate, safe choices, not to mention an opportunity to save thousands of dollars over the same treatment in their home country. Hundreds of patients who have returned from successful treatment overseas provide overwhelmingly positive feedback. They have persuaded me to write this series of impartial, scrutinizing guides to healthcare options abroad.

Why Cross Borders for Medical Care?

Cost savings. Depending upon the country and type of treatment, uninsured and underinsured patients as well as those seeking elective care can save 15–85 percent of the cost of treatment in their home country. For example, a knee surgery that costs $43,000 in the US may cost (depending on the doctors and facilities) US$12,000 abroad, including your hospital stay. The table below compares some average costs in Turkey to costs in several other countries (estimates are given in US dollars).

	Coronary Artery Bypass Graft	Heart Valve Replacement with Bypass	Hip Replacement	Knee Replacement
TURKEY**	**$11,375–15,000**	**$18,000–21,000**	**$10,750**	**$11,200**
US*	$70,000–133,000	$75,000–140,000	$33,000–57,000	$30,000–53,000
England**	$27,700	$25,000	$15,840	$20,000
Germany**	$17,335	data not available	$11,550	$11,775
Thailand*	$12,000	$17,500	$9,750	$10,000
Taiwan*	$27,500	$30,500	$8,800	$10,000
Singapore*	$16,300	$22,000	$12,000	$9,600
India*	$7,000	$9,500	$10,200	$9,200

*Source: *Patients Beyond Borders,* 2008
**Source: *Turkey: Your Partner in Healthcare.* Istanbul: DEIK Foreign Economic Relations Board, 2009
Costs are for general reference only, and vary widely. Contact hospital for exact pricing.

Better quality care. Veteran health travelers know that facilities, instrumentation, and customer service in treatment centers abroad often equal or exceed those found in their own country.

Excluded treatments. Many people don't have health insurance. Even if you do, your policy may exclude a variety of conditions and treatments. You, the policyholder, must pay these expenses out of pocket, so having the procedure in a country where it's more affordable makes economic sense.

Specialty treatments. Some procedures not available in your home country are available abroad. Some procedures that are widely practiced in certain parts of the world have not yet been approved in others, or they have been approved so recently that their availability remains spotty.

Shorter waiting periods. For decades, thousands of Canadian and British subscribers to universal, "free" healthcare plans have endured waits as long as two years for established procedures. Patients living in other countries with socialized medicine are beginning to experience longer waits as well. Some patients figure it's better to pay out of pocket to get out of pain or halt a deteriorating condition than to suffer the anxiety and frustration of waiting for a far-future appointment and other medical uncertainties.

More "inpatient-friendly." Health insurance companies apply significant pressure on hospitals to move patients out of those costly beds as quickly as possible, sometimes before they are ready. In Turkey and many other medical travel destinations, care is taken to ensure that patients are discharged only at the appropriate time and no sooner. Furthermore, staff-to-patient ratios are usually higher abroad, while hospital-borne infection rates are often lower.

The lure of the new and different. Although traveling abroad for medical care can often be challenging, many patients welcome the chance to blaze a trail, and they find the hospitality and creature comforts often offered abroad to be a welcome relief from the sterile, impersonal hospital environments so frequently encountered at home.

Safety and Security

The overriding concern of many patients new to global health travel is safety. That's understandable. Stories of wars, terrorist plots, roadside bombings, subway gassings, mad snipers, and military coups dominate the news. Obviously, we live in a troubled world. Yet, this fact remains: of the millions of patients who traveled overseas for medical treatment in the last five years, we know of no individual who has died as a result of violence or hostility.

In truth, most health travelers are usually quite sheltered. They're chauffeured from the airport to the hospital or hotel, personally driven to consultations, given their meals in their rooms, and chauffeured back to the airport when it's time to go home. US citizens who are concerned about traveling abroad can check the US Department of State's travel advisories at http://travel.state.gov/travel/cis_pa_tw/tw/tw_1764.html. Similar information services are available in other countries.

How to Use This Book

Before you dive into Part Two, please review the checklists and sidebars in **Part One, "Reminders for the Savvy, Informed Medical Traveler."** A shortened version of the more complete information in *Patients Beyond Borders: Second Edition*, it gives you some of the tools you'll need to do your research and make an informed decision. You'll find the following in Part One:

Part Two, "Turkey: A Prime Destination for the Medical Traveler," provides a brief overview of healthcare in Turkey today and profiles prominent healthcare facilities as well as several health travel agencies that serve medical travelers to Turkey. Each entry provides contact information along with a rundown on available services and history of care.

Part Three, "Turkey: A Nation to See and Love," provides details on everything from time zones to visas—basic, practical information you'll need to plan your trip. It also describes a number of the sights and experiences to be enjoyed in Turkey, and includes a handy listing of accommodations.

Part Four, "Resources and References," offers additional sources of travel information and helpful links, plus a glossary of commonly used medical terms.

As you work your way through decision-making and subsequent planning, remember that you're following in the footsteps of hundreds of thousands of health travelers who have made the journey before you. The vast majority have returned home successfully treated, with money to spare in their savings accounts. Still, the process—particularly in the early planning—can be daunting, frustrating, and even a little scary. Every health traveler I've interviewed experienced "the Big Fear" at one time or another. Healthcare abroad is not for everyone, and part of being a smart consumer is evaluating all the impartial data available before making an informed decision. If you accomplish that in reading *Patients Beyond Borders: Turkey Edition,* I've achieved my goal. Let's get started.

Reminders for the Savvy, Informed Medical Traveler

Much of the advice here in Part One is covered in greater detail in *Patients Beyond Borders: Second Edition*. Consider the following three chapters a capsule summary of essential information, sprinkled with practical advice that will help reduce the number of inevitable "gotchas" that health travelers encounter. You may want your travel companion or family members to read this section, along with the book's Introduction, so they can gain a better understanding of medical travel.

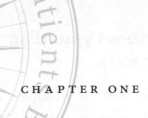

Dos and Don'ts
for the Smart Health Traveler

BEFORE YOUR TRIP

✔ *Do* plan ahead.

The farther in advance you plan, the more likely you are to get the best doctors, the lowest airfares, and the best availability and rates on hotels, particularly if you'll be traveling at peak tourist season for your destination country—in Turkey, that's June through September. If possible, begin planning at least three months prior to your expected departure date. If you're concerned about having to change plans, *do* be sure to confirm cancellation policies with airlines, hotels, and travel agents.

✔ *Do* be sure about your diagnosis and treatment needs.

The more you know about the treatment you're seeking, the easier your search for a physician will be. *Do* work closely with your local doctor or medical specialist, and make sure you obtain exact recommendations—in writing, if possible. If you lack confidence in your doctor's diagnosis, seek a second opinion.

✔ *Do* research your in-country doctor thoroughly.

This is the most important step of all. When you've narrowed your search to two or three physicians, invest some time and money in personal telephone interviews, either directly with your candidate doctors or through your health travel planning agency. *Don't* be afraid to ask questions, lots of them, until you feel comfortable that you have chosen a competent physician.

✘ *Don't* rely completely on the Internet for your research.

While it's okay to use the Web for your initial research, *don't* assume that sponsored Web sites offer complete and accurate information. Cross-check your online findings against referrals, articles in leading newspapers and magazines, word of mouth, and your health travel agent.

✔ *Do* consider traveling with a companion.

Many health travelers say they wouldn't go without a close friend or family member by their side. Your travel companion can help you every step of the way. With luck, your companion may even enjoy the trip!

✔ *Do* consider engaging a good health travel planner.

Even the most intrepid, adventurous medical traveler will benefit from the knowledge, experience, and in-country support these professionals can bring to any health journey. *Do* thoroughly research an agent before plunking down your deposit.

✔ *Do* get it in writing.

Cost estimates, appointments, recommendations, opinions, second opinions, airline and hotel arrangements—get as much as you can in writing, and *do* be sure to take all documentation with you on the plane. Email is fine, as long as you retain a written record of your key transactions. The more you get in writing, the less chance of a misunderstanding.

✔ *Do* insist on using a language you understand.

As much as many of us would like to have a better command of another language, the time to brush up on your Turkish is most definitely *not* when negotiating medical care! Establishing comfortable, reliable communication with your key contacts is paramount to your success as a health traveler. Happily for English-speaking patients, most medical staff in Turkey speak English, so communication should not be a problem.

✗ *Don't* plan your trip too tightly.

Don't plan your trip with military precision. A missed consultation or an extra two days of recovery in Turkey can mean expensive rescheduling with airlines. A good rule of thumb is to add an extra day for every five days you anticipate for consultation, treatment, and recovery.

✔ *Do* alert your bank and credit card companies.

Contact your bank and credit card companies *prior to your trip*. Inform them of your travel dates and where you will be. If you plan to use a credit card for large amounts, alert the company in advance, and reconfirm your credit limits to avoid card cancellation or unexpected rejections.

✔ *Do* learn a little about your destination.

Once you've decided on Turkey or any other health travel destination, spend a little time getting to know something about its history and geography. Buy or borrow a couple of travel guides.

Read a local newspaper. Your hosts will appreciate your knowledge and interest.

✔ *Do* inform your local doctors before you leave.

Preserve a good working relationship with your family physician and local specialists. Although they may not particularly like your traveling overseas for medical care, most doctors will respect your decision. Your local healthcare providers need to know what you're doing, so they can continue your care and treatment once you return home.

WHILE IN TURKEY
✘ *Don't* be too adventurous with local cuisine.

One sure way to get your treatment off to a bad start is to enter your clinic with even a mild case of stomach upset due to a change in water or diet. Delicious Turkish *doner kebab* and *pastirma* are best sampled after your recovery. Prior to treatment, avoid rich, spicy foods and exotic drinks. Bottled water may be safest for your stomach. During any inpatient stay, *don't* be afraid to ask the hospital's dietician for a menu that's easy on your digestion.

✘ *Don't* scrimp on lodging.

Unless your finances absolutely demand it, avoid hotels and other accommodations in the "budget" category. You *don't* want to end up in uncomfortable surroundings when you're recuperating from major surgery. On the other hand, you should be able to find a good Turkish hotel in a price range that suits you. Ask your hospital or health travel agent for a recommendation.

✘ *Don't* stay too far from your treatment center.

When booking hotel accommodations for yourself and your companion, make sure the hospital or doctor's office is nearby. Staff members at your destination hospital can advise you on suitable lodging. (Part Three provides information on lodgings near major hospitals in Turkey.)

✘ *Don't* settle for second best in treatment options.

While you can cut corners on airfare, lodging, and transportation, always insist on the very best healthcare your money can buy. Focus on quality, not just price.

✔ *Do* befriend the staff.

Nurses, nurse's aides, paramedics, receptionists, clerks, and even maintenance people are vital members of your health team! Take the time to chat with them, learn their names, inquire about their families, and perhaps proffer a small gift. Above all, treat the staff with deference and respect. When you're ready to leave the hospital, a sincere thank-you note makes a great farewell.

GOING HOME

✗ *Don't* return home too soon.

After a long flight to Istanbul or Izmir, multiple consultations with physicians and staff, and a painful and disorienting medical procedure, you might feel ready to jump on the first flight home. That's understandable but not advisable. Your body needs time to recuperate, and your in-country physician needs to track your recovery progress. As you plan your trip, ask your physician how much recovery time is advised for your particular treatment—then add a few extra days, just to be safe. You can always see some of Turkey's wonderful sights during your extra days, if you feel up to it!

✔ *Do* set aside some of your medical travel savings for a vacation.

You and your companion deserve it! If you're not able to take leisure time during your trip to Turkey, then set aside a little money for some time off after you return home, even if it's only a weekend getaway.

✔ *Do* get all your paperwork before leaving the country.

Get copies of everything. No matter how eager you are to get well and get home, make sure you have full documentation on your procedure(s), treatment(s), and followup. Get receipts for everything.

ABOVE ALL, TRUST YOUR INTUITION

Your courage and good judgment have set you on the path to medical travel. Rely on your instincts. If, for example, you feel uncomfortable with your in-country consultation, switch doctors. If you get a queasy feeling about extra or uncharted costs, don't be afraid to question them. Thousands of health travelers have beaten a well-worn path abroad, using good information and common sense. You can, too! Safe travels!

Ten "Must-Ask" Questions for Your Candidate Physician

Make the following initial inquiries, either of your health travel agent or the physician(s) you're interviewing:

1. *What are your credentials? Where did you receive your medical degree? Where was your internship? What types of continuing education workshops have you attended recently?* The right international physician either has credentials posted on the Web or will be happy to email you a complete résumé.

2. *How many patients do you see each month?* Hopefully, it's more than 50 and fewer than 500. The physician who says "I don't know" should make you suspicious. Doctors should be in touch with their customer base and have such information readily available.

3. *To what associations do you belong?* Any worthwhile physician or surgeon is a member of at least one medical association. Your practitioner should be keeping good company with others in the field.

4. *How many patients have you treated who have had my condition?* There's safety in numbers, and you'll want to know them. Find out how many procedures your intended hospital has performed. Ask how many of *your specific treatments for your specific condition* your candidate doctor has personally conducted.

5. *What are the fees for your initial consultation?* Answers will vary, and you should compare prices to those of other physicians you interview.

6. *May I call you on your cell phone before, during, and after treatment?* Most international physicians stay in close, direct contact with their patients, and cell phones are their tools of choice.

7. *What medical and personal health records do you need to assess my condition and treatment needs?* Most physicians require at least the basics: recent notes and recommendations from consultations with your local physician or specialists, x-rays or scans directly related to your condition, perhaps a medical history, and other health records. Be wary of the physician who requires no personal paperwork.

8. *Do you practice alone, or with others in a clinic or hospital?* Look for a physician who practices among a group of certified professionals with a broad range of related skills.

For surgery:

9. *Do you do the surgery yourself, or do you have assistants do the surgery?* This is one area where delegation isn't desirable. You want assurance that your procedure won't be performed by your practitioner's protégé.

10. *Are you the physician who oversees my entire treatment, including pre-surgery, surgery, prescriptions, physical therapy recommendations, and post-surgery checkups?* For larger surgical procedures, you want the designated team captain. While that's usually the surgeon, check to make sure.

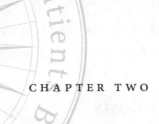

Patients Beyond Borders
Budget Planner

As with any other trip, your health travel costs will depend largely upon your tastes, lifestyle preferences, length of stay, side trips, and pocketbook. A patient flying first-class and staying at a five-star hotel can naturally expect less of a savings than one who spends frequent-flyer miles and lodges in a modest—but perfectly satisfactory—three-star hotel.

To derive an estimate of your health travel costs and savings, we suggest you use the *"Patients Beyond Borders* Budget Planner" in this chapter. Don't feel pressured to fill in every line item of your Budget Planner. Focus on the big expenses first, such as treatment and airfare, and then fill in the remainder as your planning progresses. You probably won't use all the categories. For example, you may already have an up-to-date passport, or you may stay only at a hospital and never need a hotel. The Budget Planner simply lists all the common health travel expenses. As you plan, fill in the blanks that apply to you, and you'll arrive at a rough estimate of your costs—and your savings. (You'll find more details in *Patients Beyond Borders: Second Edition*.)

A Few Notes on Costs

Passport and visa. US citizens who don't have a passport and are purchasing one for the first time should budget about $200 for fees, photographs, and shipping. Passport renewal in the US costs about $150. Passport and visa fees for other countries vary widely; check with the appropriate government office to determine Turkey's visa requirements. (See "The Medical Traveler's Essentials" in Part Three for details.)

Airfare. Air transportation will likely be your biggest non-treatment cost. It pays to shop hard for bargains. If you're okay flying coach, by all means do so; business- and first-class international travel are wildly expensive. If you have a *trusted* travel agency, use it, although with caution. Most have side deals with airlines, and their commissions and fees can cut into your savings. If you're comfortable using the Internet, take advantage of one of the many discount online travel agencies, such as Orbitz (www.orbitz.com), Expedia (www.expedia.com), Travelocity (www.travelocity.com), or CheapTickets (www.cheaptickets .com). Or go to individual airlines' Web sites, where you can sometimes snag special Internet fares. Medical travelers bound for Turkey can take advantage of an incentive program from the national air carrier, Turkish Airlines (www.turkishairlines .com), which offers significant airfare discounts to international patients and their travel companions.

International entry and exit fees. Many countries charge fees at the airport, and they may be due on arrival, on departure, or both. It's usually best to have cash in your pocket for these fees, which sometimes change dramatically without notice. At press time, Turkey was charging an airport tax of about US$20 for most arriving and departing international passengers. That cost is usually included in the price of a prepaid air travel ticket.

Rental car. When traveling, some people feel they can't manage without a car. Yet international car rentals are expensive, big-city parking is a hassle, and driving in a foreign country can land you in the hospital well ahead of your scheduled stay. It's often better for the health traveler to use taxis.

Other transportation. Transportation to and from the airport in Turkey will probably be handled by the hospital, your health travel agent, or the hotel where you or your companion will reside. Budget for the cost of transportation to and from your airport back home, and also for other transportation in Turkey. Taxis and buses are usually not expensive; US$200 should cover most two-week trips. (See Part Three for more details.)

Companions. Budget for the additional airfare and meals for your travel companion and—depending on whether you'll be doubling up—lodging. Items you can usually share include local taxi rides, mobile phone, and computer and Internet services. Items you can't share include passport and visa costs, airfare, airport fees and taxes, railway fares, meals, and entertainment.

Treatment. When you are evaluating a treatment center or physician, request the cost details in writing (email is okay), including the prices for basic treatment plus ancillaries, such as anesthesia, room fees, prescriptions, nursing services, and more. Other useful questions: Are meals included in my hospital stay? Do you supply a bed for my companion? Is there an Internet connection in the room or lobby? If you're using a health travel agency, make sure your representative gives you specific answers in writing to these important questions, along with a firm cost estimate for treatment and ancillary fees.

Lodging during treatment. These costs are straightforward and are largely a function of your tastes and pocketbook. Your doctor or your treatment center's staff can provide you with a list of preferred hotels nearby. (See "Accommodations: Recovery Lodges and Hotels" in Part Three.)

Post-treatment lodging. It's a good idea to stick around for at least a week post-treatment, because your physician will want to keep an eye on how your recovery is progressing. Many hospitals and clinics will help you arrange accommodations nearby and plan for nursing services to meet your post-treatment needs.

Meals. If you're staying in a hospital, most of your meals will probably be provided, and the food is often surprisingly good. Many hospitals offer reasonable meal plans for companions, too. Ask the facility or your agent about costs for hospital meals.

Otherwise, budget your dining out according to taste, both for you and for your companion.

Tips. Tipping customs vary widely overseas. In Turkey, it's best to tip in Turkish lira (TL), although paper money (not coins) in other currencies is acceptable. In restaurants, small tips of 5–10 percent are appreciated but not mandatory; in luxury restaurants, tip 10–15 percent. (See Part Three for more details.)

Leisure travel. Many health travelers plan a vacation for either before or after treatment. Although this expense isn't strictly a part of your health travel budget, you may want to add the costs of vacation-related lodging, transportation, meals, and other expenses into your estimated budget.

The $6,000 Rule

A good monetary barometer of whether your medical trip is financially worthwhile is the *Patients Beyond Borders* "$6,000 Rule": If your total quote for local treatment (including consultations, procedures, and hospital stay) is US$6,000 or more, you'll probably save money by traveling abroad for your care. If it's less than US$6,000, you're likely better off having your treatment at home.

The application of this rule varies, of course, depending on your financial position and lifestyle preferences. For some, a small savings might offset the hassles of travel. For others who might be traveling anyway, savings considerations are fuzzier.

Will My Health Insurance Cover My Overseas Medical Expenses?

As of this writing, it's possible, but not probable. While the largest employers and healthcare insurers—not to mention ever-vocal politicians—struggle with new models of coverage, most plans do not yet cover the costs of obtaining treatment abroad. Yet, with healthcare costs threatening to literally bust some Western economies, pressures for change are mounting. Recognizing that the globalization of healthcare is now a reality—and that developed countries are falling behind—insurers, employers, and hospitals are beginning to form partnerships with payers and providers abroad. By the time you read this book, large insurers may already be offering coverage (albeit limited) across borders. Check with your insurer for the latest on your coverage abroad.

Can I Sue?

For better or worse, many countries do not share the Western attitude toward personal and institutional liability. A full discussion of the reasons lies outside the scope of this book. Here's a good rule of thumb: if legal recourse is a primary concern in making your health travel decision, you probably shouldn't head abroad for medical treatment.

If, however, you experience severe complications and do not receive the followup care you think you need or deserve, then you may want to consider legal action, say attorneys Amanda Hayes and Natasha Bellroth of Global MD. "Legal recourse and remedies are generally limited abroad for patients who experience bad outcomes in foreign facilities," they say. "Moreover, a patient's ability to sue a foreign physician or facility for medical malpractice is limited by the availability of an appropriate forum in which to bring a lawsuit."

For example, say Hayes and Bellroth, assume that American patient John Smith travels to Istanbul for hip replacement surgery at ABC Hospital and suffers a bad outcome caused by his surgeon's negligence. Mr. Smith has some options for pursuing a judicial remedy:

✦ In order to sue ABC Hospital in the US, a US court must be able to exercise jurisdiction over ABC Hospital, a corporation in Turkey with no offices or employees in the US. US courts may only assert general or specific personal jurisdiction over a foreign entity when the foreign entity's presence or dealings where the suit is brought justify requiring the company to defend the suit there.

✦ Assuming that the case proceeds in the US to judgment against ABC Hospital, Mr. Smith faces an uphill battle to enforce an American judgment in Turkey. If Mr. Smith wins a large punitive damages award from an American court, he will be disappointed to learn that punitive damages are rarely awarded outside of the US and are unlikely to be enforced (in any of the countries currently attracting American medical travelers).

✦ Alternatively, Mr. Smith may try to sue ABC Hospital in Istanbul, which requires that he hire a lawyer in Turkey and perhaps travel back to Turkey to attend the proceedings. Even if

Mr. Smith prevails in the suit, he will probably only be able to recover his actual damages (the provable out-of-pocket cost of harm caused by negligence, e.g., medical bills incurred for corrective surgery and lost wages due to time away from work), as few countries award punitive damages to successful plaintiffs.

✦ Mr. Smith may seek to arbitrate his claim against ABC Hospital before an international tribunal. For example, the International Court of Arbitration of the International Chamber of Commerce may provide Mr. Smith with a viable and likely more cost-effective way to hold ABC Hospital accountable for negligence. Generally, an agreement to arbitrate claims must have been in place before the relationship commenced. Mr. Smith should have confirmed that prior to surgery, ABC Hospital had agreed to arbitration of potential future claims and to where those proceedings would occur.

Each alternative forum presents its own unique set of challenges. There is no ideal solution that would put judicial recourse against a foreign entity on par with the remedies available against a US hospital or physician. There are, however, practical measures that Mr. Smith might have taken before he traveled to Turkey that would have helped him manage the risk in the unlikely event of a bad outcome:

✦ For example, Mr. Smith might have purchased insurance (a health travel agency should be able to point the patient to available policies) designed specifically to protect him from the financial consequences of foreseeable complications and unforeseeable medical malpractice. Such insurance could have helped

Mr. Smith eliminate the cost of legal action while compensating him up to the amount of the policy limit he purchased.

✦ In addition, had Mr. Smith paid for his procedure with a major credit card, his card company may have allowed him to recover the cost of a disappointing treatment by disputing the charges.

✦ Finally, Mr. Smith could have made sure that his health travel agency and the treating facility had a clear and reasonable protocol in place for dealing with bad outcomes and complications. Ideally, the hospital would have agreed to absorb costs associated with making Mr. Smith whole again (return flight, accommodations, and corrective procedure) and to compensate him if he could be satisfied.

Ultimately, there is no perfect way to compensate a patient (either domestically or abroad) who has suffered an imperfect outcome after a medical procedure. The good news is that informed patients can take preventive measures to protect themselves before they travel abroad for care, so they do not end up in the hands of imperfect healthcare insurance and judicial systems.

Furthermore, foreign hospitals are eager to prove that the quality of their surgeons and technical facilities rivals or even exceeds that found in Western nations. Your independent research will reveal that sophisticated foreign hospitals and governments are heavily invested in serving international patients with high-quality healthcare; they understand that the publicity associated with even one bad outcome could quickly end the growing flow of health travelers.

Patients Beyond Borders Budget Planner

Item	Cost	Comment
IN-COUNTRY		
Passport/Visa	$200.00	For passport and visa, non-expedited
Rush charges, if any:		
Treatment Estimate		
Procedure:		
Hospital room, if extra:		Often included in treatment package
Lab work, x-rays, etc.:		
Additional consultations:		
Tips/gifts for staff:	$100.00	
Other:		
Other:		
Post-Treatment		
Recuperation lodging:		Hospital room or hotel
Physical therapy:		
Prescriptions:		
Concierge services:		Optional
Other:		
Other:		
Airfare		
You:		
Your companion:		
Other travelers:		
Airport fees:		
Other:		
Other:		
In-Country Transportation		
Taxis, buses, limos:	$200.00	
Rental car:		
Other:		
Other:		

(continued)

Patients Beyond Borders Budget Planner (*continued*)

Item	Cost	Comment
Room and Board		
Hotel:		
Food:		
Entertainment/sightseeing:		
Other:		
Other:		
"While You're Away" Costs		
Pet sitter/house sitter:		
Other:		
Other:		
IN-COUNTRY SUBTOTAL		
HOMETOWN		
Procedure:		
Lab work, x-rays, etc.:		
Hospital room, if extra:		
Additional consultations:		
Physical therapy:		
Prescriptions:		
Other:		
Other:		
HOMETOWN SUBTOTAL		
TOTAL SAVINGS:		Subtract In-Country Subtotal
		from Hometown Subtotal

Patients Beyond Borders Sample Budget Planner

Item	Cost	Comment
IN-COUNTRY		
Passport/Visa	$200.00	For passport and visa, non-expedited
Rush charges, if any:		
Treatment Estimate		
Procedure:	$9,000.00	
Hospital room, if extra:		Often included in treatment package
Lab work, x-rays, etc.:	$45.00	
Additional consultations:	$200.00	
Tips/gifts for staff:	$100.00	
Other:		
Other:		
Post-Treatment		
Recuperation lodging:	$1,100.00	Hospital room or hotel
Physical therapy:	$65.00	
Prescriptions:	$65.00	
Concierge services:	$300.00	Optional
Other:		
Other:		
Airfare		
You:	$880.00	
Your companion:	$880.00	
Other travelers:		
Airport fees:	$12.00	
Other:		
Other:		
In-Country Transportation		
Taxis, buses, limos:	$200.00	
Rental car:		
Other:		
Other:		

(continued)

Patients Beyond Borders Sample Budget Planner (*continued*)

Item	Cost	Comment
Room and Board		
Hotel:	$1,500.00	
Food:	$650.00	
Entertainment/sightseeing:	$500.00	
Other:		
Other:		
"While You're Away" Costs		
Pet sitter/house sitter:	$300.00	
Other:		
Other:		
IN-COUNTRY SUBTOTAL	$15,997.00	
HOMETOWN		
Procedure:	$55,000.00	
Lab work, x-rays, etc.:	$375.00	
Hospital room, if extra:	$4,400.00	
Additional consultations:	$1,200.00	
Physical therapy:	$400.00	
Prescriptions:	$500.00	
Other:		
Other:		
HOMETOWN SUBTOTAL	$61,875.00	
TOTAL SAVINGS:	$45,878.00	Subtract In-Country Subtotal
		from Hometown Subtotal

Your Medical Trip May Be Tax-Deductible

What do *kebabs,* taxi rides, and treatments have in common? Depending on the country you live in, these expenses may be tax-deductible as part of your health travel. In the US, for example, depending upon your income level and treatment cost, some or most of your health journey can be itemized as a straight deduction from your adjusted gross income.

In brief, if you're itemizing your deductions in the US, and if qualifying medical treatment and related expenses amount to more than 7.5 percent of adjusted gross income, the Internal Revenue Service (IRS) allows US citizens to deduct the remainder of those expenses, whether they were incurred in Toledo, Ohio, or Toledo, Spain.

For example, if a US citizen's adjusted gross income is US$90,000, then any allowed medical expense over $6,750 (7.5 percent of $90,000) becomes a straight deduction. Suppose that a medical trip costs a total of $14,000, including treatment, travel, lodging, and, of course, a two-week surgeon-recommended stay in a five-star beachfront recuperation resort; for that trip, the deduction from the US medical traveler's adjusted gross income could be $7,250 ($14,000 minus $6,750).

Of course, the expenses must be directly related to the treatment, and many specific items are disallowed. Examples of typical tax-deductible items include

- any treatment normally covered by a health insurance plan
- transportation expenses, including air, train, boat, or road travel
- lodging and in-treatment meals
- recovery hotels, surgical retreats, and recuperation resorts

Medical travelers should save all receipts and keep a detailed expense log, noting time, date, purpose, and amount paid. If you are planning to take a tax deduction, ask for letters and other documentation from your in-country healthcare provider, particularly any recommendations made for outside lodging, special diets, and other services.

For more information, US citizens can go to www.irs.gov or call 800 829.1040. Medical travelers from other countries should check their government's tax policies. It's always a good idea to consult a competent tax advisor with questions or concerns.

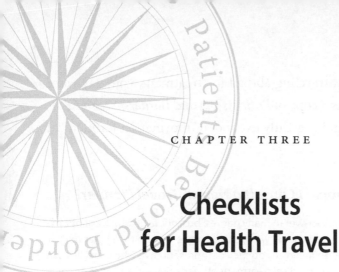

CHAPTER THREE

Checklists
for Health Travel

If you're like most readers of this book, you're *almost* sure that health travel is the right choice. You have a diagnosis and you know what medical procedure is required. You've reviewed the costs for your procedure in your home country and are beginning to believe that treatment abroad offers significant advantages— mostly financial.

But if you're like most patients contemplating medical travel, you know you have some homework to do before you get on a plane and head to a hospital or clinic abroad. While this book fo- cuses primarily on destinations for treatment in Turkey, it's a good idea to reconsider some of the questions that are relevant to all health travelers, no matter what their treatment or destination.

The seven checklists that follow will remind you of some im- portant issues and items. Review and check off those things that apply to your situation, and you'll increase your chances of a safe, happy, and healthy outcome. If you desire additional information about traveling abroad for treatment, you may want to buy or borrow a copy of *Patients Beyond Borders: Second Edition*, which contains greatly expanded information for medical travelers.

CHECKLIST 1: *Should I Consult a Health Travel Planner?*

Health travel planners answer to many names: brokers, facilitators, agents, expeditors. Throughout this book, we use the phrase "health travel planner" or "health travel agent" to mean any agency or representative who specializes in helping patients obtain medical treatment abroad. (Several agencies are profiled in Part Two.) Before engaging the services of a health travel agent, ask yourself these questions:

WHETHER TO USE A HEALTH TRAVEL PLANNER	Yes	No	Not Sure	Notes to Myself
Will a health travel planner save me time?				
Am I willing to pay for the convenience of a health travel planner's services?				
Will I feel more confident about health travel if I use the services of an agency?				
Does the agent I'm considering have the knowledge and experience I need?				
Does this planner have a track record of successful service to the health traveler?				
Does this agent speak my language well enough for us to converse comfortably?				
Can I get at least two recommendations or letters of reference from former clients of this agency? Have I checked these references?				
Can I get at least two recommendations or letters of reference from treatment centers that work with this agency? Have I checked these references?				
Can this agency give me complete information about possible destinations and options for my procedure?				

(continued)

WHETHER TO USE A HEALTH TRAVEL PLANNER	Yes	No	Not Sure	Notes to Myself
Will this agent put me in touch with one or more treatment centers and physicians?				
Will this agent work collaboratively to help me choose the best treatment option?				
Is this agent responsive to my questions and concerns?				
Does the service package this agent is offering meet my needs?				
Does this agent have longstanding affiliations with in-country treatment centers and practitioners?				
Has this planner negotiated better-than-retail rates with hospitals, clinics, physicians, hotels, and (perhaps) airlines?				
Can this agent save me money on other in-country costs, such as airport pickup and dropoff or transportation to my clinic?				
Can this agent provide personal assistance and support in my destination country?				
Is this planner willing to work within the constraints of my budget?				
Do I know (and have in writing) the exact costs for this agency's services?				
Do I have a suitable contract or letter of agreement with this agency?				
Do I feel comfortable with this agency? Have we built a sense of trust?				

When *Not* to Use a Health Travel Planner

Don't use an agent who does not promptly answer your initial requests for information, does not reasonably follow through on commitments, or does not treat you well in any way. Difficulty deciphering an agent's communications is a red flag, too. If a trusted friend or other reliable source has referred you to a specific clinic and physician, then half the work is already done, and you may want to forgo an agent's services, particularly if the hospital or clinic provides similar services (for instance, through its international patients center).

Paying for a Health Travel Planner's Services

Some planners offer "all-in-one" package deals, which are fine. However, at tax time, you may need to show your itemized cost breakdown, including treatment, lodging, meals, transportation, and health travel agent fees. Spreadsheets are universal these days. Ask your planner to give you a detailed expense log.

Costs and payments are usually handled in one of three ways:

- **Membership, upfront fee required.** This arrangement requires the patient to pay a nonrefundable membership fee (often in the US$50–300 range) before any services are rendered. The membership fee is usually folded into the package price if you engage that agent.

- **Package, advance deposit required.** In this arrangement, an agent first provides enough information to get you well along your path: data on specific treatment centers and physicians, advice on medical records and in-country procedures, and perhaps even a telephone consultation with your candidate physician or surgeon. At that point, if you decide to engage the agent, you'll be asked to submit a deposit, perhaps 25–50 percent of the entire package price. Another payment is due prior to treatment, and the remainder is payable when you leave the hospital or clinic.

- **Pay as you go, direct to third parties.** A handful of planners act more as referral services than as full-blown brokers, providing information about hospitals and physicians, airfares, and vacation opportunities, without doing much of the real legwork. They usually charge you a commission or set fee on any service you engage.

If you're dealing with a reputable agent, all these fee structures get you to much the same place. Beware, however, of agents asking for 100 percent up front. You should see evidence of performance, communicate with all the parties personally (via telephone or email), and know that your hard-earned money is going where it should.

Although a deposit of up to 50 percent of the total package cost is usually required, you should reserve at least 25 percent of the total bill for final payment. In other words, as with most other services, don't pay the entire bill until you're satisfied and all the services you were promised have been provided. Most planners accept credit cards, but before you use yours, ask your agent about any surcharges associated with credit card payments.

CHECKLIST 2: *How Can a Health Travel Planner Help Me?*

Of all the services a health travel planner offers, the most important are related to your treatment. Start your dialogue by asking the fundamental questions: Do you know the best doctors? Have you met personally with your preferred physicians and visited their clinics? Can you give me their credentials and background information? What about accommodations? Do you provide transportation to and from the airport? To and from the treatment center? If an agent is knowledgeable and capable with these details, the rest of the planning usually takes care of itself.

DOES MY HEALTH TRAVEL PLANNER PROVIDE THIS SERVICE?	Yes	No	Not Sure	Notes to Myself
Treatment options from which to choose destination countries, hospitals, and physicians best equipped to meet my needs				
Information on hospital accreditation and physicians' credentials, board affiliations, number of surgeries performed, association memberships, and ongoing training				
Appointment scheduling and confirmations for tests, consultations, and treatments				
Teleconsultation with physicians or surgeons to review my medical history and discuss my procedure				
Transfer of medical records, including history, x-rays/scans, test results, recommendations, and other documentation				
Travel arrangements, including airline and hotel reservations, tickets, and confirmations; also including local in-country transportation				
Visa or passport facilitation				
Onsite pre-treatment assistance, including a local representative to accompany me to appointments, expedite hospital admission, arrange local transportation, and assist with my hospital discharge				
Recovery arrangements, including local transportation, lodging, meals, and any nursing services required during recovery				

(continued)

DOES MY HEALTH TRAVEL PLANNER PROVIDE THIS SERVICE?	Yes	No	Not Sure	Notes to Myself
Amenity arrangements, including "concierge services," such as take-out food from restaurants, tickets for events, and dry-cleaning and laundry services				
Communications arrangements, including telephone, cell phone, and Internet services				
Leisure or vacation planning (if desired)				
Aftercare and followup once I've returned home, including post-treatment liaison for information retrieval and making arrangements for a return trip should complications arise				

CHECKLIST 3: *What Do I Need to Do Ahead of Time?*

Although each journey varies according to the traveler's preferences and pocketbook, good planning is essential to the success of any trip. That goes double for the medical traveler. This checklist covers some of the planning you'll need to do to become a fully prepared and informed global patient.

Why should you plan at least three months in advance?

- **The best physicians are also the busiest.** If you want the most qualified physician and the best care your global patient money can buy, give the doctors and treatment centers you select plenty of time to work you into their calendars.

- **The lowest international airfares go to those who book early.** Booking at least 60 days prior to treatment avoids the unhappy upward spiral of air travel costs. If you're planning to redeem frequent-flyer miles, try to book at least 90 days in advance.

- **Peak seasons can snarl the best-laid plans.** International tourism attracts large numbers of people, and you can encounter problems if you want or need to travel during the busy tourist season.

- **Everything takes longer than you think it will.** It's simply a fact of life.

For Big Surgeries, Think Big

Y ou want to be certain you're getting the best. For big surgeries, I advise heading to the big hospitals that have performed large numbers of *exactly* your kind of procedure, with the accreditation and success ratios to prove it. A hospital accredited by the Joint Commission International (JCI) carries the necessary staff, medical talent, administrative infrastructure, state-of-the-art instrumentation, and institutional followup you need. (**Note:** For more information on accreditation, see "The What and Why of JCI" and "Alternatives to JCI" below.)

Be sure to ask about the success and morbidity rates *for your particular procedure,* and find out how they compare with those at home. If you are having surgery, ask your surgeon how many surgeries *of exactly your procedure* he or she has performed in the past two years. While there are no set standards, fewer than ten is not so good. More than 50 is much better.

HAVE I COMPLETED THESE PLANNING STEPS?	Yes	No	Notes to Myself
Engaged the services of a health travel planner (if desired — see Checklists 1 and 2)			
Obtained a second opinion — or a third if necessary — on diagnosis and treatment options			
Considered a range of treatment options and discussed each option with potential providers			
Reviewed the various hospitals, clinics, specialties, and treatments available to select an appropriate destination (see Part Two)			
Chosen a reliable, fun travel companion			
Obtained and reviewed the professional credentials of two or more physicians or surgeons (see "Ten 'Must-Ask' Questions for Your Candidate Physician" in Chapter One)			
Selected the best physician or surgeon for the treatment I need			
Researched the history and accreditation of the hospital or clinic (see "The What and Why of JCI" and "Alternatives to JCI" below)			
Checked for the affiliations and partnerships of the hospital or clinic			
Learned about the number of surgeries performed in the hospital or clinic (generally, the more the better)			
Learned about success rates (these are usually calculated as a ratio of successful operations to the overall number of operations performed)			
Gathered and sent all medical records and diagnostic information that my physician or surgeon needs to plan my treatment			
Prearranged travel, accommodations, recovery, and leisure activities (if desired)			
Prearranged amenities, such as concierge services in-country or wheelchair services on the return trip			
Packed the essentials (see Checklist 4)			
Double-checked everything — then checked again			

The What and Why of JCI

When you walk into a hospital or clinic in the US and many other Western countries, chances are good that it's accredited, meaning that it's in compliance with standards and "good practices" set by an independent accreditation agency. In the US, by far the largest and most respected accreditation agency is the Joint Commission. The commission casts a wide net of evaluation for hospitals, clinics, home healthcare, ambulatory services, and a host of other healthcare facilities and services throughout the US.

Responding to a global demand for accreditation standards, in 1999 the Joint Commission launched JCI, its international affiliate accreditation agency. In order to be accredited, an international healthcare provider must meet the rigorous standards set forth by JCI. At this writing, some 240 hospitals, laboratories, and special programs outside the US have been JCI-approved, with more coming on board each month.

Although JCI accreditation is not essential, it's an important new benchmark and the only medically oriented seal of approval for international hospitals and clinics. Learning that your treatment center is JCI-approved lends a comfort to the process, and the remainder of your searching and checking need not be as rigorous. That said, many excellent hospitals, while not JCI-approved, have received local accreditation at the same levels as the world's best treatment centers.

JCI's Web site carries far more information than you'll ever want to explore on accreditation standards and procedures. To view JCI's current roster of accredited hospitals abroad, go to www.joint commissioninternational.org/JCI-Accredited-Organizations.

Alternatives to JCI

When researching hospitals and clinics abroad, you'll often come across the phrase "ISO-accredited." Based in Geneva, Switzerland, the International Organization for Standardization (ISO) is a 157-country network of national standards institutes that approves and accredits a wide range of product and service sectors worldwide, including hospitals and clinics. ISO mostly oversees facilities and administration, not healthcare procedures, practices, or methods.

Other organizations in other countries set standards and accredit hospitals. Organizations that accredit in non-JCI countries include the International Society for Quality in Healthcare, the Australian Council of Healthcare Standards, the Canadian Council on Health Services Accreditation, the Council for Health Services Accreditation of Southern Africa, the Egyptian Health Care Accreditation Organization, the Irish Health Services Accreditation Board, the Japan Council for Quality Health Care, and many more. If you are considering a hospital accredited by any organization, it's wise to investigate the criteria applied to the accreditation and determine to your own satisfaction that the standards are sufficient and appropriate to your needs.

CHECKLIST 4: *What Should I Pack?*

You've likely heard the cardinal rule of international travel: pack light. Less to carry means less to lose. Don't worry if you leave behind some basic item, such as shampoo or a comb; you can always pick it up at your destination. That said, this checklist covers the items you absolutely, positively shouldn't forget—and make sure you carry these things in your carry-on bag. A prescription or passport lost in checked luggage could spell disaster.

IS THIS ITEM PACKED IN MY CARRY-ON BAG?	Yes	No	Notes to Myself
Passport			
Visa (if required)			
Travel itinerary			
Airline tickets or eticket confirmations			
Driver's license or valid picture ID (in addition to passport)			
Health insurance card(s) or policy			
ATM card or traveler's checks			
Credit card(s)			
Enough cash for airport fees and local transportation upon arrival			
Immunization record			
Prescription medications			
Hard-to-find over-the-counter drugs			
Medical records, current x-rays/scans, consultations, and treatment notes			
All financial agreements and hard copies of email correspondence			
Phone and fax numbers, mailing addresses, and email addresses of people I need or want to contact in-country			
Phone and fax numbers, mailing addresses, and email addresses of people I need or want to contact back home			
Travel journal for notes, expense records, and receipts			

CHECKLIST 5: *What Should I Do Just Before and During My Trip?*

Now that you've made appointments with one or more physicians, booked your flights and hotel, and arranged transportation, the hard part is behind you— except, of course, for the treatment itself. You'll find that once you arrive in Turkey, you will be greeted graciously with help and support from hotel and hospital staff, your health travel agent, and sometimes even a friendly bystander. Plus, all signage at Turkey's international airports is in English, so no worries!

If you haven't done much international traveling prior to this health journey, keep in mind that you don't need to be a seasoned travel veteran to have a successful trip. Getting things done cooperatively and efficiently will help you and your companion preserve your physical *and* mental health. Knowing a little something about the culture, history, geography, and language of your host country will buy you boatloads of goodwill and appreciation. (The information in Part Three of this book will get you off to a good start.)

Tick off the items on this checklist to make sure you stay safe, happy, and well before and during your trip.

PREPARATIONS FOR MY TRIP	Yes	No	Not Sure	Notes to Myself
Have I read (or at least skimmed) a travel book or some brochures about the history, culture, and government of my destination country?				
Have I learned a few phrases, such as "please" and "thank you," in the local language?				
Have I studied a map of the city or country?				
Do I know what the local currency is, what the exchange rate is, and how I can pay for my needs in my destination country?				
Do I know the rules about the amount of cash I can carry into and out of my destination country?				
Have I found out what extra fees I will be charged for using my credit cards or ATM cards abroad?				
If I want to use traveler's checks, am I sure that my service providers will accept them? (Some don't.)				

(continued)

PREPARATIONS FOR MY TRIP	Yes	No	Not Sure	Notes to Myself
Am I leaving my valuables at home?				
If I must carry valuables, am I sure that a hotel safe or a safe-deposit box will be available to me?				
Am I prepared to drink only bottled water and eat only cooked foods? (This is a wise precaution for both the health traveler and the companion.)				
Have I packed a sanitizer for cleaning my hands everywhere I travel?				
Have I packed comfortable clothes that are sensitive to local customs of dress?				
Have I made arrangements for telephone and email services that will allow me to stay in touch with friends and relatives back home? With service providers in-country?				
Am I sure my cell phone will work in-country?				
Have I informed my doctor of all my pre-existing health conditions, such as diabetes, heart disease, ulcers, and others?				
Have I informed my physician about all prescription and over-the-counter drugs I am taking, including vitamins, minerals, and herbal supplements?				
Am I following my doctor's instructions pre-treatment, such as going off certain drugs, losing weight, or avoiding alcohol?				

Continuity of Care—Critical to Success

Continuity of care can be a challenge for patients who travel for medical procedures, say Steven Gerst, MD, and John Linss of MedicaView International (www.medicaview.com). Typically, the patient's primary physician diagnoses the condition and then suggests treatment. But when the patient chooses to travel to another location or country to receive the treatment, the primary physician is too often left out of the process.

Similarly—and amazingly—many traveling patients engage a facility to perform a procedure without speaking directly to the surgeon before arriving. The patient and the hospital's international patient services coordinator may use email for preliminary communications. There may also be a telephone call or two with the coordinator. But the surgeon may not become actively involved until the patient arrives at the facility.

Too many patients make the assumption that a diagnosis is "the end of the story" and that contact with the coordinator is all that is required. *They could not be more wrong!*

Establish Communication!

Insist on speaking to the surgeon who will perform the procedure *before* you schedule your travel. You may communicate via teleconference, videoconference, or voice over Internet protocol (VOIP).

It is equally important that you establish communication between your primary (local) doctor and your in-country surgeon, so followup care will be prearranged. Because of time zone and language differences, this advance planning may be difficult, but it is essential. Complications and misunderstandings can arise if your doctors are not communicating properly. For example, after a knee replacement or a kidney transplant, many concerns and complications can arise during the long recuperation period. Lack of communication can result in unnecessary hardships and potential returns to surgery.

Once you choose to go outside your physician's primary network, few mechanisms currently exist to encourage and facilitate ongoing consultations. *You must establish your own.* Critical information about your case can be lost if you don't. *Be proactive!* Here and abroad, it is usually up to you to keep the dialogue going between your physicians.

Persistence is important, and the time-delayed effectiveness of email comes in handy—once you get the doctors in the habit of emailing each other and you. A secure online collaboration tool is even better, because it can keep all communications in one place and available to all participants at any time.

Have Your Most Current Medical Records

Once you have established contact with a doctor (or surgeon) and facility abroad, provide them with your most current medical records. If you have a chronic condition and you've finally said "enough," your medical records may be a year or more old. If they are, visit your local physician to obtain new laboratory tests, x-rays, or scans—whatever your in-country provider needs.

Medical records can be transmitted in two ways: you can send paper copies or disks by postal service, or you can send electronic documents via a secure online service. An online service is preferable for several reasons. First, it gets the records in the hands of the surgeon more quickly. Second, it creates a secure repository that can be accessed by both your local and overseas doctors. Third and most importantly, digital records create a foundation for aftercare collaboration.

Collaboration Between Your Local Doctor and Your Doctor Abroad

Transferring your medical records may get your local doctor communicating with your in-country doctor for the first time. This communication can be achieved though email, telephone, or a private group set-up in an online environment specifically designed for that purpose. Often such an environment is part of an online repository system that provides a secure place for collaboration between the doctors via protected blog, chat, email, and VOIP. Ask your doctor or health planner if such a system is available for your destination.

The next collaboration between doctors should occur after surgery. The surgeon should notify your local physician, preferably through an online system, of the details of the surgery and the aftercare protocol.

Once you return home and are again under the care of your local physician, this collaboration and consultation should continue until you are released from care with a clean bill of health.

Complete Documentation

Frequently, when such a repository system is not utilized, patients return home lacking the complete documentation their local physician needs to oversee ongoing care. The absence of information compromises the physician's effectiveness and threatens the patient's health.

Be sure to ask the surgical facility if access is available to an electronic system of medical record-sharing and physician collaboration. If not, request that your healthcare providers abroad subscribe to one to ensure that you can keep your local physician informed.

At a minimum, make sure your in-country facility provides you with complete records when you return home. Also make sure to keep your local physician involved from the first day. Good continuity of care is essential for a successful outcome.

Remember, as a patient, you need to take responsibility for the quality and consistency of the care you receive. If you don't, no one else will!

CHECKLIST 6: *What Do I Do After My Procedure?*

You've been out of surgery for two days, you hurt all over, your digestive system is acting up, and you're running a fever. Have you somehow contracted an antibiotic-resistant staph infection? Coping with post-surgery discomfort is difficult enough when you're close to home. Lying for long hours in a hospital bed, far away from family—that's often the darkest time for a health traveler.

Knowledge is the best antidote to needless worry. As with pre-surgery preparation, ask lots of questions about post-surgery discomforts *before* heading into the operating room. Be sure to ask doctors and nurses about what kinds of discomforts to expect following your specific procedure.

If your discomfort or pain becomes acute, bleeding is persistent, or you suspect a growing infection, you may be experiencing a complication that is more serious than mere discomfort and requires immediate attention. Contact your physician without delay.

This checklist will help you make the most of your post-treatment period and know when it's appropriate to seek medical assistance.

POST-PROCEDURE PREPARATIONS AND FOLLOWUP	Yes	No	Not Sure	Notes to Myself
Have I received all my doctor's instructions for my post-treatment care and recovery? Do I understand them all?				
Am I following all of my physician's instructions *to the letter*?				
Do I know what post-treatment signs and symptoms are normal?				
Do I know what post-treatment signs and symptoms indicate a need for prompt medical attention? (See "Post-Treatment: Normal Discomfort or Something More Complicated?" below.)				
Do I have copies of all my medical records and treatment records, including x-rays/scans, photographs, blood test results, prescriptions, and others?				
Do I have itemized receipts for all the bills I have paid?				
Do I have itemized bills for all the costs I have not yet paid?				
Do I have completed insurance claim forms (if applicable)?				
Have I allotted ample time for recovery?				
Do I know how to prevent blood clots in the legs after surgery and on the airplane? (See "Caution: Blood Clots in the Veins" below.)				
Do I know what followup treatment I will need when I return home, including physical therapy?				
Have I let my family know what help I will need when I return home?				
Have I checked in with my local doctor to share information about the procedure I had and my post-treatment care needs?				
Am I staying mentally, physically, and socially active following my procedure?				

Post-Treatment: Normal Discomfort or Something More Complicated?

Prior to your surgery, your doctor should thoroughly explain the procedure and tell you about discomforts you can expect after being wheeled out of the operating unit. Discomforts differ from complications. Discomforts are predictable and unthreatening. Complications, while rarely life threatening, are more serious and may require medical attention. These are some common discomforts you can expect following surgery:

✦ minor local pain and general achiness

✦ swelling

✦ puffiness

✦ bruising, swelling, and minor bleeding around the incision

✦ headaches (side effect of anesthesia)

✦ urinary retention or difficulty urinating (side effect of anesthesia and catheters)

✦ nausea and vomiting, dry mouth, temporary memory loss, lingering tiredness (all common side effects of anesthesia)

✦ hunger and undernutrition

Most surgically induced discomforts recede or disappear altogether during the first few days after treatment, as the body and spirit return to normal. Be sure, however, to report discomforts that persist or become more pronounced, as they might be early warning signs of more serious complications.

Complications vary according to the type of surgery, and you should make sure you're aware of the more common ones. Complications are scary, and many doctors would rather not go into morbid detail about them unless pressed. Complications are rare; most arise in less than 5 percent of all cases—and generally among patients who are aged or infirm in the first place. So while it's wise to be informed and vigilant, there's no need to worry yourself sick anticipating the worst. Common symptoms of complications include the following:

✦ infection, increased pain, or swelling around the incision

✦ abnormal bleeding around the incision

✦ sudden or unexplained high fever

✦ extreme chest pain or shortness of breath

✦ extreme headache

✦ extreme difficulty urinating

If you experience any of those symptoms, call your physician immediately.

Caution: Blood Clots in the Veins

Recent surgery and the immobility of long flights increase the risk of deep vein thrombosis (DVT), which is the formation of a clot, or thrombus, in one of the deep veins, usually in the lower leg. The symptoms of DVT may include pain and redness of the skin over a vein, or swelling and tenderness in the ankle, foot, or thigh. More serious symptoms include chest pain and shortness of breath.

You can take preventive steps to reduce your risk of DVT, such as wearing compression stockings and moving about frequently when on planes and trains. Ask your doctor about how soon after surgery you can safely undertake a long, sedentary trip.

OTHER WAYS TO REDUCE DVT RISKS

Before you travel:

- Stop smoking.
- Lose weight if you need to.
- Get enough exercise to be at least minimally fit before your surgery and your travel.
- Discuss stopping birth control pills and hormone replacement therapy with your doctor.
- Travel on an airline that provides sufficient leg room.
- Wear loose clothing.
- Reserve an aisle seat on the airplane so you can get up and move around easily.
- Ask your surgeon about using a pneumatic compression device during and after surgery.
- Before your flight home, ask your surgeon if you need an anticoagulant.
- Walk briskly for at least half an hour before takeoff.

On the plane:

- Don't stow your carry-on luggage under your seat if that will restrict your movement.
- Flex your calves and rotate your ankles every 20–30 minutes.
- Walk up and down the aisle every two hours or more frequently.
- Sleep only for short periods.
- Do not take sleeping pills.
- Drink lots of water to avoid dehydration.
- Avoid alcohol, caffeine, and diet soda.
- Wear elastic flight socks or support stockings.
- Don't let your stockings or clothing roll up or constrict your legs.
- Take deep breaths frequently throughout your flight.

The Straight Dope on Pharmaceuticals

- *True or false:* When traveling, it's okay to take small amounts of prescription drugs back into your home country.
- *True or false:* It's legal to order prescription drugs from reputable online pharmacies outside your home country.

Believe it or not—for many Western countries—the answer is false on both counts, though with some favorable caveats.

Many international travelers like to purchase their prescription medications less expensively while abroad. While that's *technically* illegal in the US and some other countries, consumer activists have turned the issue into a political hot potato. Consequently, at this writing, customs inspectors in the US are often reluctant to bust granny with her two vials of benazepril, and in most instances they turn a blind eye to folks entering the country with prescription medications purchased abroad. Thus, it's become a gray area, with customs inspectors empowered to use "general discretion" when prescription drugs are found. Most often, the offending pharmaceuticals are simply confiscated, and the traveler must decide whether it's worth all the red tape required to petition for their return.

The overwhelming majority of tourists carrying pharmaceuticals purchased abroad re-enter their home country with no trouble, usually unnoticed. The best advice is to use common sense. You're far less likely to be hassled for carrying a single prescription of amoxicillin than if your suitcase is bursting with enough tramadol to supply the streets of Los Angeles for a year. And as always, if you're carrying drugs that are illegal—prescription or otherwise—you may be subject to arrest, as well as seizure of your medications.

Similarly, it's *technically* illegal in the US and some other countries to purchase any pharmaceutical of any kind from any mail-order pharmacy outside the country. Again, highly vocal activists have prevailed politically in the US and elsewhere, and only a small fraction of prescription drugs purchased from foreign pharmacies is seized. In those cases, the pharmacies often double-ship the order, so the buyer usually doesn't even know the purchase was interrupted. (It's perfectly legal to purchase prescription drugs online from authorized mail-order pharmacies inside your home country.)

Again, until the laws change, you're advised to use good judgment. Purchase only from reputable pharmacies, using legitimate prescriptions from your physician—and anticipate the outside chance you'll be among the few every year inconvenienced by border seizures of prescription drugs.

For specifics about bringing controlled substances into the US, call 202 307.2414. US citizens can obtain additional information about traveling with medication from any FDA office or by writing to the US Food and Drug Administration, Division of Import Operations and Policy, Room 12-8 (HFC-170), 5600 Fishers Lane, Rockville, MD 20857. For further information on prescription drug rules and regulations, US citizens can contact the FDA's Center for Drugs at 888 INFO.FDA or visit www.fda.gov/cder. Citizens of other countries are encouraged to contact the appropriate government office for full rules and regulations.

Taking Drugs into Turkey

Can you carry drugs into Turkey? Yes, but limit drug transport to small bottles of medications prescribed by your doctor, carried in their original, labeled vials, and accompanied by their prescriptions. Carry with you a letter signed by your doctor that explains the reason why you need a particular medication. Antidrug laws are stringent in Turkey, and penalties for possession of illicit drugs are harsh. Don't risk being stopped in customs with an unlabeled bottle of a narcotic or psychotropic substance.

CHECKLIST 7: *What Does My Travel Companion Need to Do?*

A person who accompanies a health traveler gives a great gift. Here are some questions for potential companions to answer before they commit themselves to accompanying a health traveler abroad.

TRAVEL COMPANION'S CONSIDERATIONS	Yes	No	Not Sure	Notes to Myself
Am I sure I want to go? Am I sure I'm up to the task? (If you hesitate in answering either question, you may want to reconsider.)				
Am I willing and able to take responsibility for handling details, such as obtaining visas and passports?				
Do I feel comfortable acting as an advocate for the health traveler at times when he or she may need assistance?				
Have we agreed on the costs of the trip and on who is responsible for paying what?				
Do I feel sufficiently confident about handling experiences and challenges in a foreign country, such as getting through airports, arranging for taxis, or finding addresses?				
Do the health traveler and I communicate well enough to identify problems and solve them together amicably?				
Am I prepared to listen to and record doctor's instructions and provide reminders for the health traveler when needed?				
Can I help the health traveler stay in touch with family, friends, and healthcare providers back home?				
Have I allowed for "down time" and time for myself during the medical travel?				
Do I have the patience to help the health traveler through what might be a long and difficult recovery period, both abroad and back home?				

Turkey: A Prime Destination for the Medical Traveler

Having read Part One, you now have a fair idea of what it takes to be a smart and informed health traveler. At this point, chances are you've already reached a decision about your course of treatment, and you may be seriously considering Turkey as a destination for your medical care.

Part Two gives you an overview of Turkey's developments and achievements as an international medical hub and provides in-depth information about the leading healthcare establishments, as well as health travel agents, serving medical travelers to Turkey.

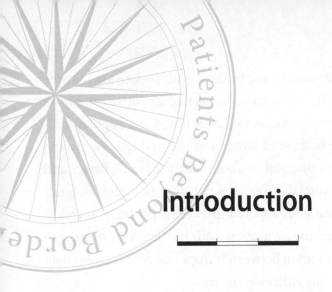

Introduction

Turkey has one foot in Europe and the other in Asia. It's an enormous country of diverse people and landscapes, ranging from the bustling commercial centers of Istanbul to the quiet agricultural villages of the eastern provinces. As a major player on the world scene both politically and economically, Turkey is poised to play its part in the global healthcare arena. With an increasing and prosperous population of 70 million, Turkey is now promoting medical travel in a big way. It is projected that Turkish medical institutions in the public and private sectors will serve 1 million foreign patients in 2015 to the tune of about US$8 billion.

Turkey has developed a booming trade in vacation tourism in the last three decades, so extending the traditional Turkish warmth and hospitality to medical travelers is not a stretch. With daily flights serving Istanbul, Ankara, and other major cities from virtually everywhere in the world, Turkey has become a magnet for medical travelers who seek competitive prices and medical excellence. Turkey is well established as a popular wellness destination because of its natural thermal spa resorts and mud baths; they alone pull in about a half-million visitors and US$100 million annually. Turkey's rich culture, beautiful landscapes, and recreational opportunities attract medical travelers who want to combine a vacation with medical treatment, and Turkey's central location between Europe and Asia is convenient for travelers heading either east or west.

The leading healthcare groups located in Turkey's three largest cities (Istanbul, Ankara, and Izmir) offer "one-stop" service to foreign patients, covering all arrangements from the day of request to the day of departure. Hoping to maximize the comfort of patients and their families, hospital staff handle everything from setting up initial consultations to booking accommodations.

As Turkey positions itself to become a full member of the European Union, the country's political, social, and economic status in the global healthcare marketplace grows. Turkey's leading healthcare providers are dedicated to promoting good health for citizens and medical travelers alike, while curbing healthcare costs. The Turkish Ministry of Culture and Tourism is now spending more than US$100 million to spread the word that Turkey is welcoming health travelers.

Turkey's Healthcare System: Among the World's Best

Lying at the crossroads between East and West, Turkey is well on its way to becoming a hub for global medical travel. According to the 2009 RNCOS report "Emerging Medical Tourism in Turkey," medical tourism in Turkey grew 40 percent from 2007 to 2008. The report asserts that cost advantages and Turkey's strategic geographic position will promote the nation's continued growth in medical travel.

Investment and Improvement

Turkey boasts 905 public hospitals, with a total bed capacity exceeding 180,000. Its private hospitals—all 308 of them—provide an additional 15,500 beds. The city of Istanbul alone offers nearly 200 hospitals and 300 clinics, collectively employing more than 100,000 people.

Healthcare accounts for 6.6 percent of Turkey's gross domestic product (compared to 13.1 percent in the US and 5.1 percent in South Korea). Recently, the number of doctors in Turkey has risen sharply, from about 29,000 in 2000 to more than 41,000 in 2006.

Health spending per capita in Turkey grew, in real terms, by an average of 5.8 percent per year between 2000 and 2005. That's one of the fastest growth rates among the countries in the Organization for Economic Cooperation and Development (OECD), and it's significantly higher than the OECD average of 4.3 percent per year. In the 1990s, Turkey was one of only two OECD countries (along with South Korea) to increase its number of acute-care hospital beds.

The Turkish pharmaceutical market grew 10 percent in 2006, reaching $9.9 billion in retail value. The market is supplied by both local production and imports. For the most part, research-based pharmaceuticals are imported or manufactured in Turkey by global producers, which include Pfizer, Novartis, Eli Lilly, Merck, and GlaxoSmithKline. Multinational firms own 14 among the 42 manufacturing facilities operating in Turkey. In the past five years, global pharmaceutical companies have bought majority shares of leading Turkish companies. Foreign companies have invested over $300 million in their local infrastructure.

Recently, Turkey has gone through a comprehensive healthcare restructuring. While the public sector accounts for approximately two-thirds of Turkey's healthcare expenditures, the greatest healthcare investment since the mid-1980s has occurred in the private sector. At that time, private investment, which had held steady at about 15 percent of the total national healthcare investment since the 1960s, started climbing sharply. In 2000 nearly 70 percent of Turkey's investment in healthcare occurred in the private sector.

Turkey's investors have raised the standards and quality of the nation's health services with an infusion of state-of-the-art treatments and medical technologies. Those investments have paid off in improvements to Turkey's healthcare—improvements that are attracting increasing numbers of medical travelers each year. For example:

✦ The delivery of healthcare services has been separated from financing.

✦ The management of public hospitals has been decentralized.

✦ The value added tax (VAT) on healthcare has dropped from 18 percent to 8 percent.

✦ Improvements are being made in healthcare infrastructure and medical technology.

✦ Specialized hospitals are opening.

✦ Turkish hospitals are collaborating with international insurance companies to offer low-cost medical care to policyholders.

In addition, Turkey's hospitals have developed affiliations and working relationships with prestigious medical centers in the US, providing opportunities for staff development, improvements in treatment, and up-to-date information exchange. Some of those affiliations include Harvard Medical International in Boston and

Johns Hopkins Medicine International in Baltimore; the Mayo Clinic in Rochester, Minnesota; Methodist Hospital in Houston; the Barbara Ann Karmanos Cancer Institute in Detroit; and in New York, the Memorial Sloan-Kettering Cancer Center, New York Presbyterian Hospital, and the university hospitals of Columbia and Cornell.

Why Medical Travelers Prefer Turkey

Few medical travelers realize that Turkey has more healthcare facilities accredited by the Joint Commission International (JCI) than any other country. Of the entire roster of JCI-accredited facilities in 36 countries around the world, Turkey boasts more than 12 percent. Its total—33 as of this writing, with new additions annually—is more than those of Thailand and India combined! Turkey's JCI-accredited hospitals offer a full range of treatments through a network of locations employing approximately 20,000 healthcare professionals, including more than 3,000 physicians.

Most travelers who go to Turkey for healthcare hail from the Middle East, the Netherlands, Germany, Azerbaijan, Albania, Georgia, Belgium, France, the UK, Sudan, Bahrain, Oman, or Kuwait. They go because prices in Turkey compare favorably with even the lowest available in Asia, and the quality of healthcare is consistently outstanding, with many doctors Western-trained and fluent in English. The Turkish government enforces rigorous quality standards in all its institutions, and healthcare is no exception. Technology, facilities, and personnel are consistently top-notch.

Patients who travel to Turkey from the Middle East, Central Asia, and the Balkan countries most often cite these three reasons for their medical travel:

✦ Medical technology and infrastructure are lacking in their home countries.

✦ Few medical colleges train doctors in their home countries, so they cannot find the professionalism and expertise they want.

✦ They don't trust the outcomes of their local medical services.

Medical travelers from Europe go to Turkey not because infrastructure and medical professionalism are lacking at home, but because waiting lists are long, important healthcare is often delayed, prices are high, and state-of-the-art technology may not be available. Also, some treatments and services are available in Turkey that cannot be obtained elsewhere. Examples include specific types of cancer treatments, organ and stem cell transplants, and assisted reproductive technologies.

No matter where they come from, medical travelers find significant cost savings in Turkey. Writing in *Medical Tourism Magazine* in 2009, David Vequist and Basak Gursoy report that the estimated cost of cataract surgery (including hospital stay and treatment) is 76 percent lower in Turkey than the average cost in the UK. The cost of rhinoplasty in Turkey runs about US$1,500, compared to US$3,500 in the UK and US$4,500 in the US. Cost savings were cited in a 2007 study as a major reason why citizens of the UK rated Turkey alongside India and Hungary as one of the top three preferred medical travel destinations in the world.

Want to Stay Up-to-Date on Medical Travel to Turkey?

The landscape of medical travel changes daily, with new hospitals and clinics gaining JCI accreditation and new specialty centers opening their doors to overseas patients. That's especially true in Turkey, where medical travel is growing rapidly. For the latest information on Turkey's newly accredited hospitals and clinics, specialty centers, treatment packages, spas, wellness weekends, recovery accommodations, and more, visit www.patientsbeyondborders .com/turkey. You'll find the latest press releases and video clips there, too.

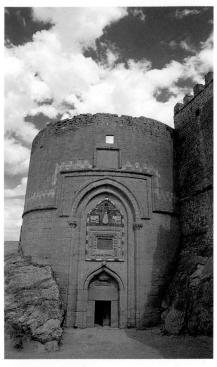

Antique City in Van

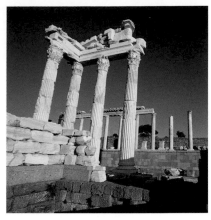

Traian Temple in Bergama

Development is
never possible
without knowing
your past.

—M. Kemal Ataturk

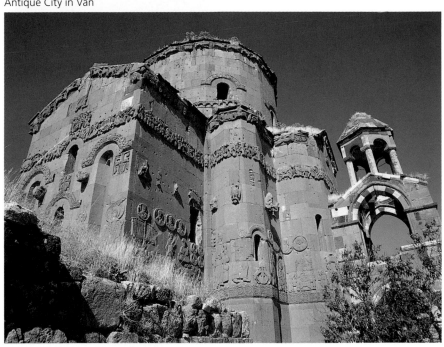

The 2,000-year-old ruins of Ani

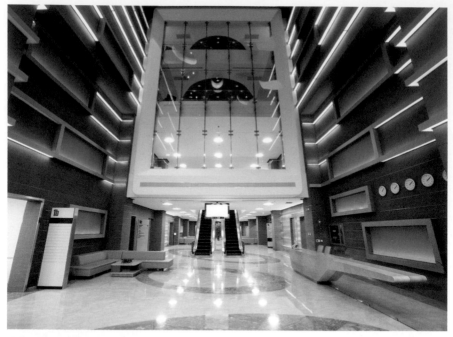

Acibadem Maslak Hospital

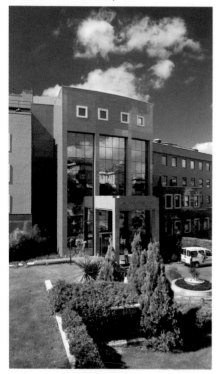

Acibadem Kadikoy Hospital

Acibadem Healthcare Group— "Passion for Excellence in Healthcare."

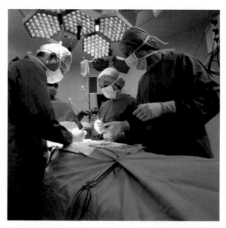

Operating theater

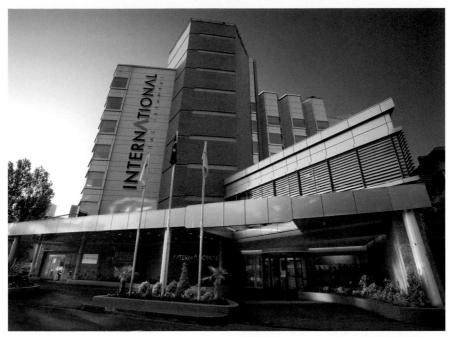

International Hospital

International Hospital—
"Where Turkish Hospitality Meets Quality and Experience."

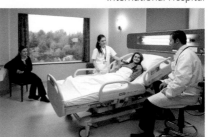

Patient rooms with sea or forest views

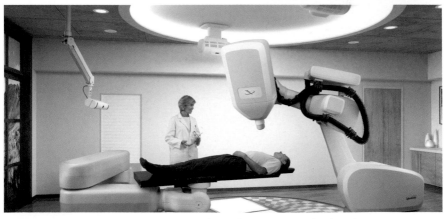

CyberKnife, the latest technology in cancer treatment

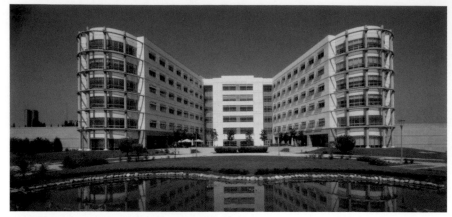

Anadolu Medical Center (AMC)

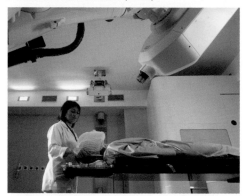

Cutting-edge treatment facilities

Anadolu Medical Center— "Advanced Healthcare with John Hopkins Medicine Expertise."

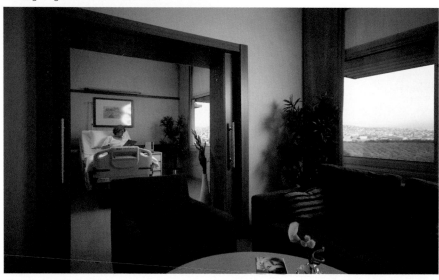

Cheerful patient suite

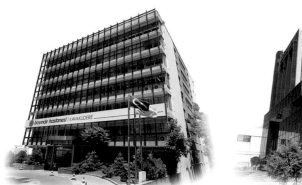

High-tech imaging equipment

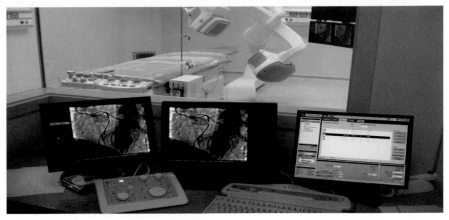

Bayindir Hospital Kavaklidere

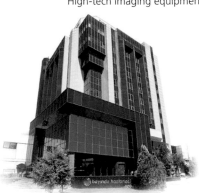

Bayindir Hospital Sogutozu

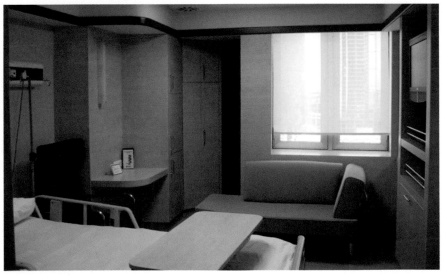

Modern patient room

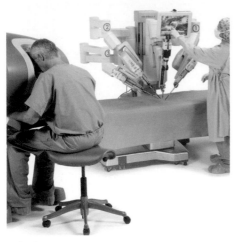

Robotic surgery

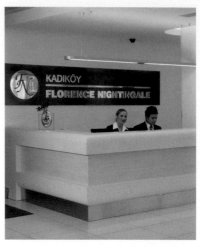

Admissions desk

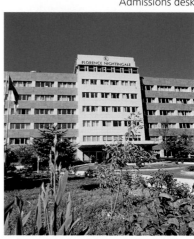

Sisli Florence Nightingale Hospital

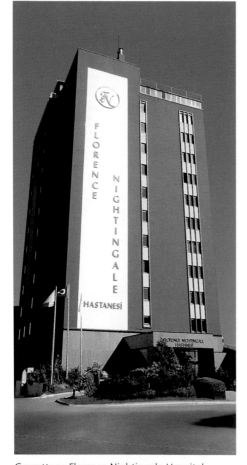

Gayrettepe Florence Nightingale Hospital

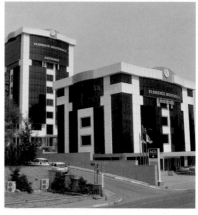

Kadikoy Florence Nightingale Hospital

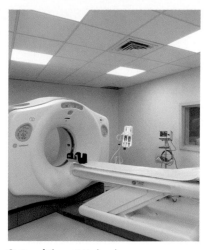

State-of-the-art technology

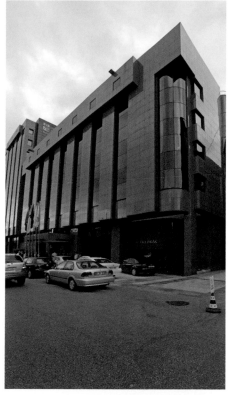

Ankara Guven Hospital is located in the core of Ankara, in the center of the embassy region.

Ankara Guven Hospital

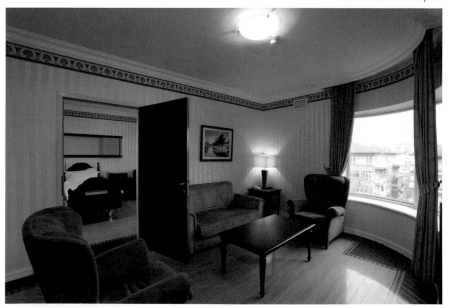

The comfort and safety of "smart-room" design

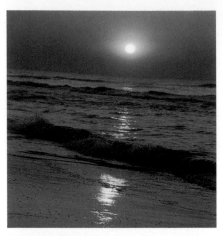

A Mediterranean sea view

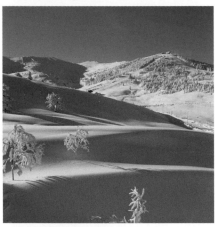

Uludag Mountain, Bursa

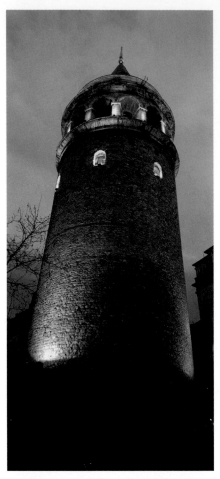

The ancient Galata Tower

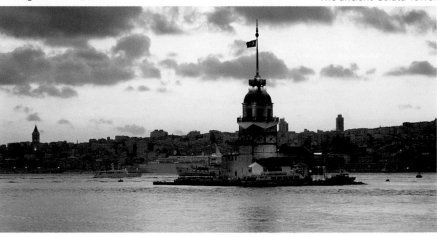

The Maiden Tower in Istanbul

Specialties That Attract Medical Travelers to Turkey

Patients travel to Turkey from Europe, Russia, the Balkan countries, the Middle East, and Central Asia seeking specialized healthcare that is unavailable, inadequate, or prohibitively expensive at home. This section reviews the medical specialties that most often attract medical travelers to Turkey.

Bone Marrow Transplantation

Bone marrow transplantation (BMT) is a specific type of hematopoietic stem cell transplantation. It is most often performed for patients who have diseases of the blood and bone marrow or certain types of cancers, including leukemia, lymphoma, and multiple myeloma. BMT can be used for children with such congenital conditions as aplastic anemia, severe combined immunodeficiency, congenital neutropenia with defective stem cells, and thalassemia. Other conditions treated with BMT include

Ewing's sarcoma, Hodgkin's disease, myelodysplastic syndrome, neuroblastoma, and sickle cell disease. These transplants may be autologous (using the patient's own stem cells) or allogeneic (from a healthy, tissue-matched donor).

Cardiology and Cardiovascular Surgery

Turkish hospitals provide the full range of cardiology services, from examination and diagnosis through intervention, intensive care, and rehabilitation. Diagnostic procedures include computed tomography (CT), echocardiography, electrocardiography (EKG), and magnetic resonance imaging (MRI). New 2×64 multislice CT scanners enable instant diagnosis with a higher-quality outcome than conventional diagnostic modalities, including angiography. In 2008 Turkish surgeons performed more than 10,000 cardiovascular surgeries, and more than 30,000 interventional cardiology cases were treated in Turkey's leading accredited hospitals. Minimally invasive techniques can be applied to bypass surgery, coronary angioplasty, and stent implantation. Complex coronary bypass surgeries are performed on the beating heart with the help of the Impella micropump device, utilized in Turkish hospitals since 2008. The Heart Turcica cardiac pump is currently being developed and tested in Turkish medical research centers.

Dentistry

In Turkey's dental facilities, techniques for the preservation, restoration, and replacement of teeth include bonding, dentures, extraction, implants, and porcelain veneers. Turkish dentists provide complete dental implant services, from planning to surgery to final restoration, as well as cosmetic and general dentistry.

Genetics

Turkish hospitals offer a wide range of genetic tests. In addition to clinical sample testing, advanced research is being conducted in gene therapy to combat a range of medical problems, from malignant tumors to the adverse effects of organ transplantation.

Neurosurgery

Turkish specialists in adult and pediatric neurosurgery treat cancers of the brain and nervous system, degenerative spinal disorders, disc disease, hydrocephalus, vascular disease of the brain and spinal cord, and more. Multidisciplinary teams perform functional neurosurgery, neuroendoscopy, and peripheral nerve surgery. All three types of epileptic surgery (disconnection, resection, and vagal nerve stimulation) are available. Turkey's leading private hospitals have become regional and international referral centers for Gamma Knife and CyberKnife treatments, and Istanbul boasts the world's first operating theater to use an internal 3-Tesla MRI scanner.

Obstetrics and Gynecology and Assisted Reproduction

The obstetrics and gynecology departments of Turkey's JCI-accredited hospitals offer international patients several sought-after subspecialties. Fertility diagnosis (including determination of the partner's sperm count), intracytoplasmic sperm injection (ICSI), and in vitro fertilization (IVF) are commonly conducted. Prenatal diagnostic tests include amniocentesis, chorionic villus sampling, fetal blood sampling, first-trimester screening, maternal serum screening, and more. Gynecological status and ovulatory condition are evaluated thoroughly in treating such medical problems as endometriosis, polycystic ovarian disease, and tubal disorders. Surgeries are performed for gynecological cancer patients.

Oncology

Every year Turkey's leading private and accredited hospitals perform thousands of medical oncology treatments as well as major, complex oncological surgeries. Providing both early diagnosis and treatment for cancer, Turkish healthcare institutions take a multidisciplinary approach to combat tumors, using biotherapy, chemotherapy, immunotherapy, radiotherapy, surgery, and more. Treatment can be delivered orally, systemically, or directly at the tumor site. Turkish physicians use radiosurgical CyberKnife and Gamma Knife treatments as appropriate. Other specialized techniques employed include image-guided radiation therapy (IGRT), intensity-modulated radiation therapy (IMRT), and three-dimensional conformal radiotherapy, as well as RapidArc, brachytherapy, and ultrasound-guided transperineal prostate implantation of isotopes.

Ophthalmology

Ophthalmology departments in Turkish healthcare facilities use advanced technology to perform a broad range of eye surgeries. LASIK surgeries have attracted international patients to Turkey for many years, because complications are rare and prices are low. In cases unsuited for laser surgery, Intacs (for keratoconus) or phakic intraocular lens implants may be utilized. Medical and surgical treatments for glaucoma and disorders of the cornea and retina are often performed at Turkey's JCI-accredited hospitals.

Orthopedics and Traumatology

Another strength of Turkey's healthcare is treatment for a wide range of orthopedic diseases and musculoskeletal impairments. The orthopedics and traumatology branches in Turkish hospitals are staffed with experts in numerous subdisciplines, including musculoskeletal oncology. Orthopedic physicians and surgeons specialize in pediatric care as well as the treatment of spine, shoulder, knee, hip, hand, and foot injuries in adults. A very new treatment, free vascularized fibula grafting for extensive knee osteonecrosis, is now available in Turkey. Turkish physicians and therapists are also internationally recognized for their expertise in the management of athletic injuries. All procedures are complemented by post-surgery physical therapy and rehabilitation.

Plastic Surgery

Turkey's most frequently performed aesthetic and plastic surgeries are abdominoplasty ("tummy tuck"), armlift, and mammoplasty (breast augmentation or reduction); browlift, cheekbone and chin augmentation, eyelid surgery, facelift, necklift, and rhinoplasty ("nose job"); fat transfer and liposuction; genital surgery; and reconstructive surgery in oncology cases. Plastic surgeons offer a variety of individualized services, including endoscopic aesthetic surgery and facial rejuvenation with fat cell transfer. Nonsurgical aesthetic treatments, such as Botox injections, are also available.

Transplantation

Transplantation can provide hope for some patients suffering from end-stage organ failure. Turkey's first organ transplant took place in 1969, and since then the expertise of Turkish doctors and the infrastructure for organ transplantation have both grown rapidly. Surgeons in Turkey specialize in bone, kidney, liver, pancreas, and stem cell transplantation. Organ transplants for kidney and liver cases are frequently performed from live donors. At the Ninth Meeting of the Turkish Transplantation Society in 2007, distinguished physicians from around the world convened to exchange knowledge and insights on the current state of research, new techniques, and future directions.

In Istanbul in 2008, the participants at the International Summit on Transplant Tourism and Organ Trafficking drafted and signed "The Declaration of Istanbul on Organ Trafficking and Transplant Tourism," establishing stringent ethical standards governing the circumstances under which nonresidents can obtain a transplant within a given country. These guidelines are followed scrupulously within Turkey to ensure that every transplant conducted is legal, ethical, and morally defensible.

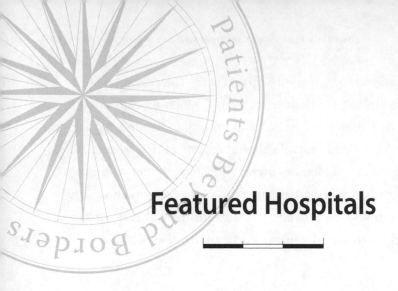

Featured Hospitals

Acibadem Healthcare Group

Altunizade Mah.
Fahrettin Kerim Gokay Cad. 49
Uskudar
Istanbul, TURKEY 34662
Tel: 90 216 544.3981
Fax: 90 216 340.7710
Email: international@asg.com.tr
Web: www.acibademinternational.com;
www.acibadem.com.tr/English

Acibadem Healthcare Group offers integrated health services through a 25-branch network of hospitals, medical centers, outpatient clinics, and more (see the following sidebar). The network comprises a total of 73 operating rooms, 1,367 beds, and more than 8,500 employees, including 1,580 physicians. Acibadem Healthcare Group is Turkey's largest private healthcare network, and provides 10% of all private services in Istanbul.

Members of Acibadem Healthcare Group

Acibadem Healthcare Group has facilities in Istanbul, Kocaeli, Bursa, Adana, and Kayseri. As of this writing, the group boasts six hospitals accredited by the Joint Commission International (JCI). Four of them—Bakirkoy, Kadikoy, Kozyatagi, and International—are located in Istanbul, all within 10–30 minutes driving distance from a major aiport. The other two are equally convenient: Acibadem's Kocaeli Hospital (30 minutes from Istanbul's Sabiha Gokcen International Airport) and Acibadem Bursa Hospital, which is located in one of Turkey's most-visited tourist spots.

While JCI is now accrediting only individual hospitals, from 2005 to 2008, Acibadem was the first and only hospital network to be accredited as a system. Acibadem has applied for JCI accreditation for its other member hospitals, among them the Adana, Kayseri, and Maslak facilities. Readers are encouraged to check the JCI Web site, www.joint commissioninternational.org/JCI-Accredited-Organizations/#Turkey, for the most recent updates on Acibadem's JCI accreditations, as well as any other newly accredited hospitals in Turkey.

Acibadem's other medical centers and clinics include the following: Acibadem Beylikduzu Medical Center, Acibadem Bagdat Outpatient Clinic, Acibadem Etiler Outpatient Clinic, Acibadem Uludag Outpatient Clinic (located at a ski center popular among Europeans), and the International Etiler Outpatient Clinic. The group has widened its service network in recent years with Acibadem Central Laboratories, Acibadem Insurance Company, Acibadem Project Management, A-Plus catering and laundry services, Acibadem Mobile ambulance service, and Acibadem University.

The group's ongoing projects include Acibadem Bodrum Hospital (located in a popular tourist town), Acibadem Eskisehir Hospital, and Acibadem Fulya Hospital, which has plans to become a major facility for orthopedics, traumatology, and sports medicine.

Acibadem prides itself on its state-of-the-art technologies. It was the first healthcare group in Turkey to acquire a 3-Tesla intraoperative MRI scanner, which enables many types of tumor surgeries to be performed with a high success rate. For cancer treatment, Acibadem boasts nine linear accelerators and was also Turkey's first private healthcare group to acquire a Gamma Knife, which delivers a precisely targeted dose of radiation to tumor sites. The latest addition to its radiosurgical infrastructure is the CyberKnife, used for many previously untreatable cancers. Acibadem has also accumulated extensive experience in robotic surgery and in the use of intensity-modulated radiotherapy (IMRT), image-guided radiotherapy (IGRT), and RapidArc. All medical data and images are electronically stored and accessed through a picture archiving and communications system (PACS).

Acibadem's wide variety of specialty centers includes units focused on **Arrhythmia, Bone Marrow Transplantation, Breast Disease, Genetic Diagnosis and Cord Blood Bank, Hair Transplantation, Hepatobiliary Surgery, High-Risk Pregnancy, IVF, Microsurgery, Movement Disorders, Neonatal Intensive Care, Obesity, Pain, Pre-implantation Genetic Diagnosis, Spasticity,** and **Stroke.**

In 2003 Acibadem signed a partnership agreement with Harvard Medical International to promote high-level professional development of the network's doctors, nurses, and other clinical staff. Additionally, Acibadem enjoys a cooperative relationship with Massachusetts General Hospital in the development of software programs for advanced MRI technology. The group has also fostered relationships with international insurance companies and assistance companies.

Acibadem's **International Patient Center** offers comprehensive, compassionate service and support to meet the unique needs and expectations of medical travelers and their families. Within 48 hours of a treatment inquiry, the center's staff responds with a treatment plan, estimated length of stay, and average package pricing that incorporates all medical, accommodation, and ancillary costs.

Specialties

✦ Cardiology and cardiovascular surgery (adult and pediatric)

✦ Dentistry

✦ Dermatology

✦ Ear, nose, and throat

✦ Emergency medicine

✦ General surgery

✦ Internal medicine

✦ Neurology and neurosurgery (adult and pediatric)

✦ Nuclear medicine

✦ Obstetrics and gynecology

✦ Oncology (adult and pediatric)

✦ Ophthalmology (adult and pediatric)

✦ Orthopedics (including spinal surgery)

✦ Pathology

✦ Pediatrics and pediatric surgery

+ Physical therapy and medical rehabilitation

+ Plastic and reconstructive surgery

+ Radiology and interventional radiology

+ Radiosurgery and radiotherapy

+ Reproductive medicine and infertility

+ Thoracic surgery

+ Urology

Services Provided for International Patients

+ Appointment scheduling, including pre-operative and post-operative evaluation

+ Visa assistance

+ Flight reservation and confirmation assistance

+ Assistance with international insurance

+ Accommodations arrangement

+ Airport pickup and dropoff

+ Land and air ambulance services

+ Assistance to patient and family before, during, and after hospitalization

+ Assistance with admission and discharge

+ Multilanguage interpretation

+ Assistance with financial arrangements and transactions

+ Liaison with medical tourism agents, employers, and insurance companies

+ Assistance with local tours and excursions

Achievements and Awards

✦ 1991: Turkey's first healthcare group to offer helicopter ambulance services

✦ 2000: First healthcare organization traded on the Istanbul Stock Exchange

✦ 2002: Turkey's first healthcare group approved by the Ministry of Education to open an academic university, the Acibadem Education and Healthcare Foundation

✦ 2002: Turkey's first healthcare group to establish a Genetic Diagnosis Center and Cord Blood Bank

✦ 2002: European Foundation for Quality Management (EFQM) membership

✦ 2003: Harvard Medical International affiliation

✦ 2003: Turkey's first digital radiology and paperless hospital

✦ 2004: EFQM Commitment to Excellence Award

✦ 2004: World's first 3-Tesla intraoperative MRI

✦ 2005: Noted by *Turkishtime* magazine for largest number of teaching physicians

✦ 2006: European Board of Nuclear Medicine admittance

✦ 2006: Noted by Nielsen research as best-known brand in Turkey's healthcare industry

✦ 2007: Named "Fastest Fish of Turkey" by *Referans* newspaper for investment success among 1,300 companies in 54 cities

Feature Story

Surgeons at Acibadem Bakirkoy Hospital Correct Anomalies in a Boy's Heart

Approximately half of all children born with Down's syndrome also have congenital heart anomalies. In the case of three-year-old James Larsen, his mother reports that his condition was not diagnosed prenatally. "When our baby was born, we learned that he had Down's syndrome. We were very surprised. Two days after his birth, the doctors detected abnormal sounds in his heart. Echocardiography was done, and his heart problem was discovered," she says.

Medical records and images of the child's heart were sent to hospitals in the US and the UK. "All the doctors who analyzed the results stated that the problem was very complex," says James's mother, who is a doctor at Emirates International Hospital in Dubai. The physicians of Harvard Medical International/Dubai Healthcare City referred the Larsen family to Acibadem Healthcare Group. Despite being a US citizen with treatment opportunities in other countries, Dr. Larsen chose Acibadem Bakirkoy Hospital for her son.

Dr. Tayyar Sarioglu, head of the cardiovascular department at Acibadem Bakirkoy's Cardiac Center, found two major defects in James's heart: a tetralogy of Fallot (a cluster of four heart abnormalities) and an atrioventricular block (a failure of the heart contraction signal to pass properly from its upper to its lower chambers). During a six-hour operation, in which the child's heart was stopped for an hour and a half, Dr. Sarioglu repaired eight malfunctions: a defect between the atria, a defect between the ventricles, right and left heart valve disease, an opposite vascular outlet, stenosis of the right outflow tract, closure of the vascular shunt, and vascular stenosis of the lung.

After a short period in intensive care, James recovered quickly and completely. "The surgery went even better than we expected," his mother says. "The hospital took great care of my son. I am honored he was treated in a hospital in Turkey with such good facilities. The close attention we received made us very happy. Although I knew that the surgery was risky, I was quite comfortable at Acibadem." Dr. Sarioglu, reporting on the success of the surgery, emphasized that such procedures can be conducted only in centers combining extensive experience and advanced technology.

Now back home in Dubai, James is attending nursery school and continuing his music lessons. His mother says, "If the problems in his heart had not been corrected, he would have been unable to engage in such activities. We owe his life to these doctors."

Anadolu Medical Center (Anadolu Foundation)

Anadolu Cad. No. 1
Bayramoglu Cikisi
Cayirova Mevkii, Gebze
Istanbul, TURKEY 41400
Tel: 90 262 678.5513
Fax: 90 262 654.0053
Email: int.patients@anadolusaglik.org
Web: www.anadolumedicalcenter.org

Operating since 2005, Anadolu Medical Center (AMC) is a JCI-accredited hospital with more than 200 physicians and surgeons, 209 beds, eight operating rooms, and a large intensive care unit. Through its affiliation with Johns Hopkins Medicine International, AMC's multilingual nurses and staff members receive training from the Johns Hopkins faculty. AMC physicians are commonly US-trained and US board–certified. The medical center's 42-acre (17-hectare) campus is home to treatment facilities, medical offices, and health-related retail stores—all well away from the hustle and bustle of Istanbul. The campus has earned praise for its architecture and location atop a hill bordered by woodlands and olive groves, a man-made pond, and a spectacular sea view. Outreach services are also provided at two satellite clinics in Istanbul (AMC Atasehir and AMC Suadiye).

AMC prides itself on its marriage of cutting-edge technology with a hospitable, patient-friendly environment. The hospital was the fourth in Europe to use CyberKnife, the latest radiosurgery technology, which delivers precise high-dose radiation to tumors (see AMC's "Feature Story"). Linear accelerators with an IMRT system are also available for cancer treatment, and a new **Bone Marrow Transplantation Unit** was added in 2009, making AMC an international oncology referral center. The hospital utilizes state-of-the-art imaging technology, PACS, telemedicine, and electronic recordkeeping.

AMC offers many medical specialties and subspecialties, with procedures ranging from bariatric surgery and deep brain stimulation to pediatric cardiac surgery and comprehensive, personalized health screenings. The hospital also engages multidisciplinary teams of physicians to resolve complicated health problems. The **Tumor Board,** for instance, concentrates on precise cancer diagnosis and effective treatment; other teams address back pain, cardiac arrhythmia, diabetes, stroke, and more.

For patients, physicians, and referring organizations seeking an objective assessment of available treatment options, the hospital provides a **Medical Second Opinion Program, Diagnosis Confirmation Program,** and **Telemedicine Program.**

International patients can have their cases reevaluated by AMC's specialists without traveling outside of their home country. After receiving the medical data by email, fax, or regular mail, the AMC physicians review the case and typically return a treatment plan and cost estimations within 24–48 hours. A high-tech video conferencing system enables collaboration with consulting physicians from other countries.

Each year AMC's **International Patient Services Department** facilitates more than 3,000 medical visits by patients from more than 60 countries. The department's staff members answer questions and handle all arrangements, from medical consultations to the hospital stay. AMC provides free transportation from airports to local hotels and to medical appointments and treatment facilities. (Sabiha Gokcen International is the closest airport, located approximately 15 minutes away. Ataturk International Airport, on the European side of Istanbul, is about an hour away.) If arrangements are made in advance, VIP transportation service can be provided for patients and their traveling companions.

Patients and patients' families visiting AMC are welcome to stay at its on-campus guesthouse, comprising 29 standard rooms, two handicapped-access rooms, eight suites, and one executive suite.

International patients can exchange currency and complete financial transactions at the hospital's onsite bank; its ATM allows withdrawals for Visa, MasterCard, Union Pay, and American Express cardholders. Patients can pay for healthcare services with cash, credit, or bank transfer. AMC also works with a large number of insurance and assistance companies worldwide.

Specialties

✛ Aesthetic/cosmetic and reconstructive surgery

✛ Alzheimer's disease

✛ Bariatric surgery

✛ Bone marrow transplantation

✛ Cardiology and cardiovascular surgery and therapy (adult and pediatric)

✛ Dentistry

✛ Dermatology

✛ Diabetes

✛ Endocrinology

✛ Epileptology

✛ General surgery

✛ Interventional radiology

✛ Hand surgery and microsurgery

✛ Health checkups

✛ Hematology

✛ Intensive care

✛ IVF and reproductive health

✛ Maxillofacial surgery

✛ Minimally invasive surgery

✛ Neurology and neurosurgery (adult and pediatric)

✛ Nuclear medicine

✦ Oncology

✦ Ophthalmology

✦ Orthopedics, traumatology, and sports medicine

✦ Otolaryngology

✦ Pain management/algology

✦ Pediatric nephrology

✦ Physical therapy and rehabilitation

✦ Radiosurgery and radiotherapy

✦ Rheumatology

✦ Stroke

✦ Urology

Services Provided for International Patients

✦ Appointment scheduling

✦ Telemedicine communications (for diagnosis confirmation or second opinion)

✦ Travel arrangements

✦ Accommodations arrangement (onsite, hotel, or long-term lodging) for patients and families

✦ Airport pickup and local transportation

✦ Land and air ambulance transportation

✦ Assistance before, during, and after hospitalization

✦ Direct admission

✦ Personal escort to appointments and procedures

✦ Private-duty nursing

✦ Interpretation in 30 languages

✦ Special meals accommodating cultural needs

✦ Secretarial services

✦ Business center with Internet access and cable television

✦ Amenities including on-campus pharmacy, hairdresser, supermarket, gift shop, and free wi-fi

✦ Liaison with assistance organizations and insurance companies

✦ Concierge services for shopping, dining, sightseeing, and Istanbul-area events

Achievements and Awards

✦ 2005–2015: Affiliation with Johns Hopkins Medicine International

✦ 2005 and 2007: JCI accreditation

✦ 2006–2007: Recognized by Canada's Operational Support Command for high-quality healthcare provided to the Canadian Intermediate Staging Team while in Turkey

✦ 2007: European Society for Medical Oncology Certification as a Designated Center of Integrated Oncology and Palliative Care

Feature Story

An Englishman's CyberKnife Treatment at Anadolu Medical Center

In 2007 John Stuart, then 66 years old, underwent a number of tests to determine the cause of his stomach problems. In 2008 he had an operation to bypass his bile duct, and his surgeon took a biopsy of Stuart's pancreas. A week later, Stuart received a diagnosis of pancreatic cancer.

"The tumor was inoperable," Stuart says. "My [doctor] told me that I had three to four months to live, but it could be a bit longer with chemotherapy. I was wiped out momentarily, because I wasn't expecting it."

Two months after his diagnosis, Stuart read a newspaper article about CyberKnife treatment. "After reading the article, I immediately started looking into this treatment. I was surprised to see that it was not available in the United Kingdom."

Through his research, Stuart learned that the CyberKnife Robotic Radiosurgery System is a noninvasive alternative to surgery for cancers of the prostate, lung, brain, spine, liver, kidney, and pancreas. CyberKnife delivers beams of high-dose radiation to the tumor site with extreme accuracy, a treatment option that appealed to Stuart, as the precise targeting of the radiation poses a lesser risk of killing healthy tissue.

After considering several hospitals, Stuart contacted a medical travel agent, who arranged for him to receive CyberKnife treatment at Anadolu Medical Center. After a first trip to Turkey for the implantation of radioactive markers in his tumor, he subsequently returned to AMC for three two-hour CyberKnife sessions—a painless procedure, according to Stuart. Several months later, he returned once more to AMC, where scans determined that his tumor had shrunk.

Stuart says, "[At] Anadolu Medical Center . . . patients are given utmost attention. The care provided is exceptional. All doctors, nurses, and personnel are extraordinary, very welcoming and comforting. Anadolu Medical Center provided me with the care [I needed]."

Ankara Guven Hospital

Simsek Sok. No. 29
Kavaklidere
Ankara, TURKEY 06450
Tel: 90 312 457.2525
Fax: 90 312 468.8030
Email: guven@guven.com.tr
Web: www.guven.com.tr

Ankara Guven Hospital was the first private hospital to be established in Ankara as well as in the entire Near Anatolian region. The Kucukel family founded the hospital in 1974 and has been operating it ever since. Today Guven is a 387,500-square-foot (36,000-square-meter) facility with 163 beds and eight operating rooms. It boasts up-to-date medical technologies and a modern hospital infrastructure, with computer-controlled systems and a 150-person seminar room for staff development courses and training sessions.

Examination, diagnosis, surgical intervention, and specialized care are provided at Guven around the clock, seven days a week. The hospital's medical staff comprises 130 physicians (40 percent of whom also have academic titles), 248 nurses, and 110 allied health professionals, including audiologists, dieticians, emergency technicians, pharmacists, physiotherapists, and more.

Guven became JCI-accredited in 2008 and provides services in all specialties. Along with its emergency department and general intensive care unit, the hospital has specialized intensive care facilities for newborns and cardiovascular patients. Guven's specialty centers also include the **Atherosclerosis Center, Dementia Center, Dermatocosmetology Center,**

Diabetics Club, Menopause Center, and **Smoking Cessation Center.**

Approximately 150,000 patients are treated at Guven every year: 35,000 in the emergency department, 95,000 as outpatients, and 20,000 admitted as inpatients. Annually, its surgeons and physicians perform nearly 2,000 cardiovascular surgeries (coronary bypass graft, valve operations), 1,700 general surgeries (breast surgery, gastroenterological surgery, thyroidectomy), 1,000 gynecological surgeries, 1,000 orthopedic surgeries, and 1,500 deliveries. The hospital treats about 4,500 international patients each year; in 2008 more than 600 patients visited Guven from the US and Canada alone.

Specialties

✦ Cardiology and cardiovascular surgery

✦ Dermatocosmetology

✦ Diabetes

✦ Ear, nose, and throat

✦ Emergency medicine

✦ Endocrinology

✦ Gastroenterology and gastroenterological surgery

✦ General surgery

✦ Geriatric medicine

✦ Hematology

✦ Intensive care

✦ Internal medicine

✦ IVF

✦ Nephrology

✦ Neurology and neurosurgery (adult and pediatric)

✦ Nuclear medicine

✦ Obstetrics and gynecology

✦ Ophthalmology

✦ Orthopedics and traumatology

✦ Pediatrics

✦ Physical therapy and rehabilitation

✦ Plastic and reconstructive surgery

✦ Radiology

✦ Respiratory medicine

✦ Thoracic surgery

✦ Urology

✦ Vascular surgery

Services Provided for International Patients

✦ Appointment scheduling

✦ Flight reservations

✦ Accommodations arrangement

✦ Airport pickup

✦ Assistance before, during, and after hospitalization

✦ Language interpretation: English, French, German, Italian, and Russian

Achievements and Awards

✦ 2005 to present: White House Medical Unit Certificates of Appreciation

✦ 2007: United Kingdom Accreditation Service certification

✦ 2007: German Association for Accreditation and German Accreditation Council certifications

✦ 2008: JCI accreditation

Feature Story

Heart Surgery at Ankara Guven Hospital for a Man from Azerbaijan

In February 2009, Ankara Guven Hospital received an inquiry about treatment for a 69-year-old citizen of Azerbaijan who had been diagnosed with atherosclerotic heart disease, chronic obstructive lung disease, hypertension, and diabetes. Guven's Cardiology-Cardiovascular Surgery Council evaluated the patient's history and approved his admission to the hospital, and a representative of the hospital's Foreign Patient Department made arrangements for his air transport and accommodations.

On the day of his arrival at Guven, the patient underwent a battery of diagnostic tests, including coronary angiography. The angiogram revealed obstructions measuring 100 percent in his left anterior descending artery, 70 percent in his circumflex artery, and 95 percent in his right coronary artery. The next day, he underwent coronary bypass graft surgery using the beating-heart technique. He was transferred from the coronary intensive care unit the following day to begin recovery in the cardiovascular surgery unit. Discharged from the hospital only nine days after he'd arrived, the patient continued followup monitoring and treatment with his cardiovascular surgeons, endocrinologist, diabetes nurse, and respiratory physiotherapists.

After his experience at Guven, he sent a letter to the hospital:

I am writing to express my sincere appreciation for the outstanding care that your hospital recently provided to me. Your staff's attention to details and consistent attempts to make my stay as comfortable as possible made what could have been a very stressful event more manageable. Dr. Haldun Karagoz and his team provided outstanding care and answered all questions and concerns both prior to and following my operation. I would especially like to note the assistance provided by the Foreign Patient Department staff. Their caring attitude and positive approach were a great comfort to me and my family throughout the whole process.

Bayindir HealthCare Group

Bayindir Hospital Kavaklidere

Ataturk Bulv. No. 201
Kavaklidere
Ankara, TURKEY 06680
Tel: 90 312 428.0808
Fax: 90 312 428.0629
Email: ipk@bayindirhastanesi.com.tr
Web: www.bayindirhastanesi.com.tr

One of two hospitals operated by Bayindir in Ankara, Bayindir Hospital Kavaklidere opened its doors in 1998. This 22-bed facility has two operating rooms, a three-bed intensive care unit, and 24-hour emergency services, as well as full-time laboratory and radiology units. The hospital currently employs 32 physicians, nine surgeons, and 135 additional staff members—nearly all speak English, and some speak French, German, and Russian, too. Bayindir Kavaklidere is best known for its departments of obstetrics and gynecology, ocular health and disease, oral and dental health and disease, and physical therapy and rehabilitation. Head and neck surgeries are also frequently performed, as are adult allergy testing, dermatocosmetic procedures, and gastrointestinal endoscopy.

Specialties

✦ Allergy

✦ Cardiology

✦ Dermatology

✦ Ear, nose, and throat

✦ Emergency medicine

✦ Endocrinology and metabolic medicine

✦ General surgery

✦ Head and neck surgery

✦ Intensive care

✦ Internal medicine

✦ Neurology and neurosurgery

✦ Obstetrics and gynecology

✦ Ophthalmology

✦ Oral and dental medicine

✦ Orthopedics and traumatology

✦ Pediatrics

✦ Physical therapy and rehabilitation

✦ Radiology

✦ Respiratory medicine

✦ Urology

Bayindir Hospital Sogutozu

Kizilirmak Mah. 53
Cad. No. 2
Sogutozu
Ankara, TURKEY 06520
Tel: 90 312 287.9000
Fax: 90 312 285.0733
Email: ipk@bayindirhastanesi.com.tr
Web: www.bayindirhastanesi.com.tr

Bayindir Hospital Sogutozu earned JCI accreditation in 2006. Part of Ankara's healthcare sector since 1992, this 169-bed hospital is only a ten-minute drive from the heart of the city. It employs 98 physicians and surgeons and nearly 600 additional staff. The facilities include an outpatient clinic, emergency room, diagnostic and medical imaging center, medical laboratory units, and comfortable rooms for patients. Six modular operating rooms, equipped with a laminar airflow system to lower the risk of infection, are used for all types of surgery. The hospital's 35-bed intensive care unit is equipped with the most modern life-support systems available.

One of Bayindir Sogutozu's premier centers is its **Department of Cardiology and Cardiovascular Surgery.** The array of noninvasive tests offered include color Doppler echocardiography, EKG and exercise EKG, Holter monitoring, and 24-hour blood pressure monitoring; invasive procedures include coronary angiography and angioplasty (balloon stent atherectomy), left/right heart catheterization, and mitral and pulmonary valvuloplasty. The department's open-heart surgical procedures include aneurysm repair, coronary bypass surgery, correction of congenital defects, and valve replacement and repair. Closed-heart procedures are also conducted, including constricted mitral valve commissurotomy, pericardiectomy, and shunt operations. Vascular surgery is performed to treat carotid artery defects, disorders of the large abdominal and thoracic vessels, and peripheral vascular disease.

Bayindir Sogutozu is also well known for its departments of general surgery, head and neck surgery, obstetrics and gynecology, and orthopedics and traumatology. Other frequently performed procedures include gastrointestinal endoscopy, interventional radiology (peripheral angiography and vascular and nonvascular procedures), and pediatric allergy testing.

Specialties

✦ Allergy

✦ Cardiology and cardiovascular surgery

✦ Dermatology

✦ Ear, nose, and throat

✦ Endocrinology and metabolic medicine

✦ Gastrointestinal disease and endoscopy

✦ General surgery

✦ Head and neck surgery

✦ Internal medicine

✦ Neurology and neurosurgery

✦ Nuclear medicine

✦ Obstetrics and gynecology

✦ Ophthalmology

✦ Orthopedics and traumatology

✦ Pediatrics and pediatric surgery

✦ Physical therapy and rehabilitation

✦ Radiology and interventional radiology

✦ Respiratory medicine

✦ Thoracic surgery

✦ Urology

✦ Vascular surgery

Feature Story

Unexpected Orthopedic Surgeries for Two Tourists at Bayindir Hospital Sogutozu

Australians Michael Gardiner, 65, and Joanna Krygier, 64, traveled to Turkey in December of 2008—and wound up in a car accident in Cappadocia. They both suffered serious injuries in the accident and were admitted to Bayindir Hospital Sogutozu, where evaluation determined that spinal surgery was required in both cases.

Orthopedic specialist Dr. Oguz Okan Karaeminogullari performed a minimally invasive kyphoplasty on Gardiner. In this operation, a balloon is inflated in the spine to expand a collapsed vertebra, and the space thus created is filled with a bone-cement mixture to restore the bone's structure and strength. Dr. Karaeminogullari also performed a posterior instrumentation stabilization and fusion on Krygier. This operation bonds vertebrae together to prevent motion in the affected part of the spine, with a rod holding the bones in position until the fusion can heal.

Following their successful surgeries and a 22-day stay in the hospital, both patients were discharged from Bayindir Sogutozu in 2009. After their return to Australia, they sent a letter to their healthcare providers back in Turkey:

Dear Dr. Oguz, Dr. Murat, Dr. Indy, and All Your Colleagues,
Both Doctors and Nurses,

Sorry it has taken so long for us to contact you, but we have been very busy with people visiting us. We found an excellent orthopedic surgeon [here], Michael Ryan, who looked at [our records] and said that you did a great job....

We tell our family and friends how unbelievably lucky we were to have arrived at your hospital with wonderful doctors and nurses. We were so well looked after. We miss your visits ... when we almost always managed to laugh about something.

Most of all, we want to thank you again for your thoughtfulness and kindness, which made our stay in the hospital a most pleasurable experience which we shall never forget.

Warmest wishes,
Joanna and Michael

Florence Nightingale Group

The Florence Nightingale Group traces its history back to 1989, when Sisli Florence Nightingale Hospital was established under the auspices of the Turkish Cardiology Foundation. Three other hospitals have since been added to the group: Gayrettepe Florence Nightingale Hospital in 1997, and Kadikoy Florence Nightingale Hospital and Gokturk Florence Nightingale Medical Center in 2007. Sisli, Gayrettepe, and Kadikoy are accredited by JCI.

The Florence Nightingale hospitals share radiological and other diagnostic images using the newest PACS technology. Fully equipped meeting centers enable participation in international conferences and hosting of meetings via direct satellite connections. Collectively, the group collaborates with several world-renowned medical schools and hospitals, including

✦ Barbara Ann Karmanos Cancer Institute, Detroit

✦ Baylor College of Medicine, Houston

✦ Center for Cell Therapy and Cancer Immunotherapy, Tel Aviv

✦ Columbia University Medical Center, New York

✦ Detroit Medical Center, Detroit

✦ Memorial Sloan-Kettering Cancer Center, New York

✦ Methodist Hospital, Houston

✦ Wayne State University School of Medicine, Detroit

✦ Weill Medical College of Cornell University, New York

International Patients at Florence Nightingale Hospitals

The **International Patient Department** of any hospital in the Florence Nightingale Group can be contacted through a shared inquiry system:

Tel: 90 212 224.4984

Fax: 90 212 296.5220

Email: international@florence.com.tr

Web: www.florence.com.tr; www.groupflorencenightingale.com

Services Provided for International Patients

- International medical services Web site
- Appointment scheduling
- Accommodations arrangement
- Language interpretation
- Assistance before, during, and after hospitalization
- Direct admission
- Medical referrals
- Communication with evaluation agents, employers, and insurance companies

Gayrettepe Florence Nightingale Hospital

Gayrettepe Mah.
Cemil Aslan Guder Sok. No. 8
Besiktas
Istanbul, TURKEY 34349
Tel: 90 212 288.3400
Fax: 90 212 288.9812
Web: www.florence.com.tr; www.groupflorencenightingale.com

Gayrettepe Florence Nightingale Hospital was first JCI-accredited in 2003 and earned reaccreditation in 2006. This 100-bed hospital offers inpatient and outpatient diagnosis and treatment facilities that include a fully equipped radiology department. Its six operating suites are used for a wide variety of procedures, from laser cataract removal to microlaparoscopy to prostate surgery. The hospital's specialties include gynecology, IVF, oncology, and plastic surgery.

Gayrettepe employs a wide range of imaging technologies, including digital angiography, mammography, 2×64 multislice CT, MRI, positron emission tomography (PET)-CT, ultrasound, x-ray, and more. The **Nuclear Medicine Unit** and **Nuclear Cardiology Unit** also use a Gamma Camera (for example, to determine the extent of damage from myocardial infarction).

Three types of patient rooms are available, all featuring ergonomic and orthopedic beds, satellite television, telephone, and private bath.

Gayrettepe's centers of excellence include

✦ **In Vitro Fertilization Unit and Infertility Treatment Unit,** providing a full range of assisted reproduction services, from preimplantation genetic diagnosis to embryo freezing. In addition to classical IVF and microinjection, these units offer testicular sperm extraction (TESE) and aspiration (TESA), epididymal sperm aspiration (ESA), and microsurgical and percutaneous epididymal sperm aspiration (MESA and PESA).

✦ **Oncology Center,** offering comprehensive, integrated medical and surgical oncology, chemotherapy, and radiotherapy. IMRT is used to deliver higher levels of irradiation to cancerous tissue while avoiding healthy tissue. For some lung cancer cases, the **Bronchoscopy Unit** provides radiotherapy from inside the lung, a practice thought to shorten the treatment period, enhance treatment effectiveness, and reduce problems stemming from radiotherapy. This center works in cooperation with leading cancer centers worldwide, including the Barbara Ann Karmanos Cancer Institute (Detroit), the Center for Cell Therapy and Cancer Immunotherapy (Tel Aviv), and Memorial Sloan-Kettering Cancer Center (New York).

✦ **Robotic Surgery in Urology Unit,** utilizing the da Vinci Robotic Surgical System to perform prostatectomies.

Kadikoy Florence Nightingale Hospital

Bagdat Cad. No. 63
Kiziltoprak, Kadikoy
Istanbul, TURKEY 34724
Tel: 90 216 450.0303
Fax: 90 216 450.1950
Web: www.florence.com.tr; www.groupflorencenightingale.com

Kadikoy Florence Nightingale Hospital entered service in 2007 and attained JCI accreditation in 2009. The 74-bed hospital provides inpatient and outpatient services in all specialties. Among its facilities are diagnostic units, fully equipped radiology and angiography departments, a flat-detector x-ray system, treatment and emergency facilities, and several polyclinics.

Kadikoy's centers of excellence include

✦ **Cardiology and Cardiovascular Surgery Center,** a polyclinic rendering services with modern technologies that include blood pressure and Holter monitoring, echocardiography, and treadmill testing. Angiography and bypass surgery are performed.

✦ **Physical Therapy and Rehabilitation Center,** treating muscular and skeletal diseases, including rheumatoid arthritis and osteoarthritis, herniated discs, neck and back pain, sports injuries, and various problems in shoulders, elbows, hips, knees, and ankles.

✦ **Plastic Surgery Center,** performing aesthetic surgery for obesity, breast reduction and replacement surgery, nose and facial reconstruction, and more.

Sisli Florence Nightingale Hospital

Abide-i Hurriyet Cad. No. 290
Sisli
Istanbul, TURKEY 34403
Tel: 90 212 224.4950
Fax: 90 212 224.4982
Web: www.florence.com.tr; www.groupflorencenightingale.com

When Sisli Florence Nightingale Hospital opened in 1989, it had a capacity of only 50 patient beds and performed only 250 open-heart surgeries annually. Today it operates as the largest private hospital in Turkey, where some 2,500 heart surgeries and 3,500 general surgeries are performed each year. State-of-the-art diagnostic technologies at Sisli include a 3-Tesla MRI scanner and a multislice CT scanner for angiography. The hospital was first JCI-accredited in 2004 and earned reaccreditation in 2007.

Sisli's centers of excellence include

✦ **Cardiology and Cardiovascular Surgery-Angiography and Rhythm Disorders Center,** with a 35-member surgical staff treating patients in 12 operating rooms and three procedure rooms. Over the last 20 years, Sisli has performed about 40,000 heart surgeries and 100,000 angiography, balloon angioplasty, coronary laser, permanent pacemaker, and stent procedures.

✦ **Organ Transplantation Center,** in which 30 doctors, nurses, and technicians perform about 100 kidney and liver transplants annually (from both living and cadaver donors). The team also carries out studies on biliary tract, liver, and pancreatic diseases; removes tumors of the liver and pancreas; and treats tumors with radiofrequency ablation (RFA) when appropriate.

✦ **Plastic Surgery Center,** where specialists perform aesthetic surgery for obesity, breast reduction and replacement, and nose and facial reconstruction.

Feature Story

Cosmetic Surgery at Kadikoy Florence Nightingale Hospital Helps a Woman to Improve Her Life

Nikole was a 27-year-old woman living in Switzerland. After graduating from a public relations course in 2005, she sent her résumé to several well-known institutions over the next two years—but although she was well trained and knowledgeable in her field, she did not obtain employment at any of them.

Nikole feared that her appearance and speech were holding her back professionally, as she had a large, deviated nose, which caused breathing trouble and made her voice sound strange. Additionally, she felt that her small breasts were affecting her private life; for example, she lacked the self-confidence to go swimming with her boyfriend because of her small bust size.

Wanting to make some positive changes in her life, she mentioned her concerns to a friend, who suggested that she contact Dr. Hasan Findik, a specialist in aesthetic, plastic, and reconstructive surgery at Kadikoy Florence Nightingale Hospital. After getting in touch with Dr. Findik, Nikole then traveled to Turkey to meet him, and subsequently underwent rhinoplasty and breast implant surgery at the hospital.

After the operations, Nikole found increased personal and professional happiness. She is now working in her chosen career at a prestigious organization.

Hisar Intercontinental Hospital

Alemdag Cad.
Site Yolu No. 7
Umraniye
Istanbul, TURKEY 34768
Tel: 90 216 524.1300
Fax: 90 216 524.1357
Email: mozsoy@hisarhospital.com
Web: www.hisarhospital.com

Opened in 2005, Hisar Intercontinental Hospital is the first health investment of Hisar A.S., a developing firm in the fields of training, research, and medical device marketing. This 111-bed private hospital employs more than 80 physicians and surgeons and about 400 other staff, who provide outpatient and inpatient services in a building with the largest indoor area among hospitals in Turkey. It received JCI accreditation in 2007.

Hisar Intercontinental's specialized facilities include a hyperbaric oxygen treatment unit, which is the first and only one housed in a private hospital in Turkey. The hospital also features seven operating rooms and numerous intensive care beds: 19 general and cardiovascular, six coronary, eight intermediate, and eight neonatal.

Hisar Intercontinental prides itself on its intelligent building technology, such as the two synchronous generators and uninterruptible power supplies that guarantee continuous electricity for the hospital's many high-tech electronic and computer-controlled systems. A digital imaging system with high-resolution screens in the operating rooms enables surgical teams to analyze and follow angiography, CT, MRI, and x-ray images as needed during surgery. Through a wireless telemetry system, patients moving freely inside and outside the hospital can be monitored for vital indicators, such as EKG and blood oxygenation. A computerized medication management system ensures administration of the correct drug to the correct patient, at the correct time, in the correct dose.

Located near new residential areas and modern business centers on Istanbul's Asian side, Hisar Intercontinental is easily accessible from Istanbul's ring roads and both Bosphorus bridges, and is a 15-minute drive from the European side of the city. It's also within easy traveling distance from Sabiha Gokcen International Airport, which is 15 minutes away on the Asian side of Istanbul, and from Ataturk International Airport, 40 minutes away on the European side.

Hisar Intercontinental's centers of excellence include

✦ **Cardiology and Cardiovascular Surgery Department,** utilizing an EKG management system (the first in Turkey) and three-dimensional echocardiography for diagnosis and treatment monitoring. An implantable cardioverter defibrillator may be employed in patients at risk for ventricular tachycardia or fibrillation. Frequently performed procedures include beating heart bypass, cardiac valvular operations, pediatric cardiac operations, and vascular surgery.

✦ **Eye Health and Diseases Department,** where a wavefront system is utilized to deliver fast, accurate diagnosis. The department provides precise, individualized treatment for the broadest range of visual imperfections, with diagnostic information linked to the appropriate laser treatment. Wave-front-guided LASIK is used for the correction of myopic and hyperopic disorders and mixed astigmatism. Laser instrumentation with an iris-recognition system is also used. With an IntraLase femtosecond laser, surgeons achieve a more predictable flap thickness, better astigmatic neutrality, and decreased epithelial injury after LASIK. Another frequent procedure in this department is "cold phaco," which employs ultrasound to break up cataracts.

✦ **Hyperbaric Oxygen Treatment Unit,** especially effective for nonhealing wounds (diabetic and nondiabetic) and chronic infections. Hyperbaric oxygen therapy can also achieve dramatic improvement in several other conditions, such as air and gas embolisms, anoxic encephalopathy, brain abscess, carbon monoxide poisoning, decompression sickness, compartment syndrome, crush injuries, excessive blood loss, other traumatic circulatory disorders, radiation injuries, thermal burns, and sudden hearing loss.

✦ **Plastic and Reconstructive Surgery Department,** also offering hand surgery and microsurgical operations. This department's most frequently performed cosmetic procedures include facelift, liposuction, mammoplasty, and rhinoplasty. Reconstructive and restorative surgery is conducted to correct congenital anomalies and repair burn injuries.

✦ **Radiology Department,** one of the leading neuroradiological imaging centers in Turkey. Aneurysms, cerebral hemorrhage, and cerebrospinal vascular disease are treated with endovascular methods. Service is provided using MRI-compatible anesthesia devices and followup monitoring. Radiological images are stored and transmitted by means of PACS and remote installation services.

✦ **Urology Department,** offering extracorporeal shock wave lithotripsy (ESWL) as a specialized treatment for kidney stones. Perfect focusing is achieved using an Inline Focusing System. (Patients who have lung and heart disorders can be treated with ESWL by using linked EKG.)

Specialties

✦ Cardiology and cardiovascular surgery (adult and pediatric)

✦ Hand surgery

✦ Hyperbaric oxygen therapy

✦ Intensive care

✦ Microsurgery

✦ Ophthalmology

✦ Pediatric surgery

✦ Plastic and reconstructive surgery

✦ Radiology, interventional radiology, and neuroradiology

✦ Urology

Services Provided for International Patients

✦ Air ambulance transfer of emergency cases to the hospital's heliport

✦ Airport pickup and dropoff for patients and their families

✦ Assistance with arrangements for hotel accommodations and city tours

✦ Package prices

✦ Information on followup care

✦ Language interpretation

✦ Patient rooms equivalent to five-star hotel rooms, with in-room multimedia entertainment system and Internet access

✦ Separate rooms for patients' companions

✦ Webcam/Internet communications for patients and their relatives

✦ Electronic transfer of patient data, medical records, and followup care instruction

✦ Assistance with administrative and financial matters (such as bank remittances and foreign exchange transactions)

✦ Arrangements with foreign assistance companies to offer patients payment choices

Achievements and Awards

✦ 2006: Eko-Star Hospital Quality Award

✦ 2007: World Health Organization (WHO) Baby-Friendly Hospital designation

✦ 2009: *Hospital Magazine* Sponsorship Award

Feature Story

Hisar Intercontinental Hospital's Surgeons Save a Man's Legs

Arzuman Musayev of Azerbaijan suffered from circulatory system disease due to diabetes and cigarette smoking. He had previously sought help at medical centers in Germany, where he had been told that the way to save his life was to amputate both legs at the knee level. Seeking an alternative to amputation, he was admitted to Hisar Intercontinental Hospital in July 2007.

At Hisar Intercontinental, Musayev was examined by cardiovascular surgeons, who chose a different treatment approach and subsequently performed peripheral vascular bypass surgery. In this surgical technique, blood flow to the legs and feet is rerouted from above a blocked portion of an artery to another blood vessel below the obstruction. The specific bypass procedure is named for both the artery that is bypassed and the artery that receives the rerouted blood flow. In Musayev's case, two procedures were necessary: an aortobifemoral bypass, which directs blood from the aorta in the abdomen to the two femoral arteries in the groin; and a femoropopliteal bypass, which directs blood from the femoral artery to the popliteal arteries above or below the knee.

This surgery saved the man's legs—only the tips of his toes had to be amputated. Following his operation, Musayev received treatment at Hisar Intercontinental's in-hospital hyperbaric oxygen facility, and he recovered well. Before returning home, he expressed his gratitude to the hospital staff.

International Hospital

Istanbul Cad. No. 82
Yesilkoy
Istanbul, TURKEY 34149
Tel: 90 212 468.4444; International Call Center 90 212 444.0663
Fax: 90 212 663.2862
Email: international@asg.com.tr
Web: www.internationalhospital.com.tr

Since its establishment in 1989, International Hospital has achieved many firsts in medical technologies and applications. It was the first private hospital in Turkey to offer open-heart surgery, neonatal intensive care, an IVF center, sea ambulance service, an intensive-care-equipped land ambulance, diagnostic MRI scanning, PET scanning, and an image-transfer system. After joining Acibadem Healthcare Group in 2005, International Hospital earned JCI accreditation in 2008. One-quarter of its nearly 900 physicians are also faculty members at Acibadem University and other educational institutions.

International Hospital is best known for aesthetic/cosmetic and reconstructive surgery, assisted reproductive medicine, invasive cardiology, neurosurgery (adult and pediatric), and obstetrics and gynecology. It is also well known for its pediatrics department, in which subspecialists—such as hematologists, oncologists, cardiologists, and rheumatologists—collaborate closely to ensure children's health and well-being. The procedures most frequently performed in International Hospital's six operating theaters are brain tumor surgery, coronary artery bypass surgery, and hip and knee replacement. The specialized facilities in this 134-bed hospital include a 12-bed general intensive care unit, a six-bed coronary intensive care unit, a nine-bed heart surgery intensive care unit, six neonatal intensive care incubators, seven hemodialysis beds, an angiography laboratory, and nine emergency room beds. The intensive care units (all single-patient) were designed in accordance with the latest international standards of function, patient safety, and confidentiality.

Patients at International Hospital stay in single rooms complete with a bathroom, minibar, telephone, cable television, folding bed for a companion, and a view of the Sea of Marmara. Renovations in 2007–2008 updated the entire hospital's infrastructure, medical technology, and patient care areas. Through its **International Patient Center,** the hospital treats approximately 300 international patients annually, including about 50 medical travelers from the US and Canada. The **International Call Center** operates 24/7 and handles about 150,000 inquiries per month.

Specialties

Diagnostic

✦ Audiology

✦ Cardiology

✦ Clinical laboratory

✦ Electroencephalography (EEG) and electromyography (EMG)

✦ Endoscopy

✦ Nuclear medicine

✦ Pulmonary function testing

✦ Radiology

✦ Surgical pathology

✦ Urology

Clinical

✦ Cardiology and cardiovascular surgery

✦ Dentistry

✦ Dermatology

✦ Ear, nose, and throat

✦ General surgery

✦ Health checkups

✦ Hemodialysis

✦ Infectious disease

✦ Intensive care

✦ Internal medicine

✦ IVF and assisted reproductive medicine

✦ Neurology and neurosurgery (adult and pediatric)

✦ Nuclear medicine

✦ Obstetrics and gynecology

✦ Ophthalmology

✦ Orthopedics and traumatology

✦ Pediatrics and pediatric surgery

✦ Physical therapy and rehabilitation

✦ Plastic and reconstructive surgery

✦ Respiratory medicine

✦ Speech-language pathology

✦ Thoracic surgery

✦ Urology

Services Provided for International Patients

✦ Appointment scheduling, including pre-operative and post-operative evaluation

✦ E-consultation

✦ Visa assistance

✦ Accommodations arrangement

✦ Airport pickup and dropoff arrangement

✦ Assistance to the patient and family before and after arrival

✦ Assistance with hospital admission and discharge

✦ Language interpretation (Albanian, Arabic, Bulgarian, English, French, German, Italian, Persian, Russian, and Spanish)

✦ Assistance with international insurance

✦ Assistance with payment procedures and financial transactions

✦ Local tour and excursion arrangement

✦ Daily delivery of international publications

✦ Satellite television (US, UK, and other European channels)

✦ Free wireless Internet access throughout the hospital

Achievements and Awards

✦ 1989: Turkey's first neonatal intensive care unit

✦ 1990: Turkey's first private hospital to offer open-heart surgery

✦ 1990: Turkey's first in vitro fertilization center

✦ 1993: Turkey's first sea ambulance

✦ 1994: Turkey's first MRI center

✦ 1994: Japanese Overseas Health Administration Center designation as Center for Healthcare

✦ 1997: Turkey's first intensive-care-equipped ambulance

✦ 1997: Turkey's first image-transfer system

✦ 1998: WHO Baby-Friendly Hospital designation

✦ 2000: Turkey's first PET scanner

✦ 2008: White House Medical Unit Certificates of Appreciation

Feature Story

Treatment for an Albanian Burn Victim at International Hospital

Adriana Cullaj was the quality-control inspector at an alcohol factory in Albania. One day she and her assistant were checking some containers hidden in deep shadow, and her assistant held a flashlight so they could see them—but he accidentally dropped it. A spark set fire to some alcohol (possibly leakage on the floor), and Adriana found herself surrounded by a ball of flame.

"I began to run fast," she says. "I could feel the flames on my back and on my legs. I entered an empty room. When I looked at myself, my legs, feet, and arms were burned. I had severe pain." Adriana was taken to a hospital, where doctors determined that she had severe burns over 40 percent of her body.

"The doctors in Albania said that there was nothing that could be done. They said I was going to die," Adriana says. Her employer came to the hospital as soon as he heard about the accident. He had previously received treatment at International Hospital in Istanbul, so he called his doctors there and arranged for Adriana's transportation to Istanbul via air ambulance.

At International, Adriana was a patient in the intensive care unit for a month and underwent ten operations. Her wounds were frequently cleaned and dressed, and her body was carefully protected from infection. As her treatment progressed, the burned areas were repaired with skin patches. Because of the burns, Adriana's body faced serious challenges in its protein and water balance, but her caregivers worked tirelessly to restore her health.

Adriana reports that the doctors and nurses at International were very kind to her—"The nurses complimented me every morning, saying 'You're very pretty' and 'You're like a flower'"—and were eager to see improvement in her life-threatening condition. "My doctors were saying that I would be like I was before, and they gave me moral support." Adriana recovered fully, and says, "I owe my life to the doctors and nurses who cured my burns and wounds."

Istanbul Memorial Hospital (Memorial Healthcare Group)

Piyale Pasa Bulv.
Okmeydani, Sisli
Istanbul, TURKEY 34385
Tel: 90 212 314.6666
Fax: 90 212 314.6667
Email: internationalpatients@memorial.com.tr
Web: www.memorial.com.tr

Memorial Healthcare Group opened Istanbul Memorial Hospital in 2000, and in 2002 the hospital became Turkey's first JCI-accredited healthcare institution. This 216-bed facility (including 42 intensive care beds) now has a staff of 160 physicians, many of them trained in the US or Europe, and recently made a large investment in the complete technological renovation of its radiology department with cutting-edge equipment. Memorial also offers its own five-star guesthouse, with eight single and two double suites, to recovering patients and their families.

In the international healthcare arena, Memorial is best known for cardiovascular surgery, gastroenterology, orthopedics and traumatology, IVF, and organ transplantation, specifically kidney, pancreas, liver, and intestine. The hospital treated more than 5,000 international patients in 2008, most of them from the Balkans, Germany, Italy, Middle Asia, the Netherlands, and the US.

In 2004 Memorial became Turkey's first private hospital licensed by the Ministry of Health to carry out organ transplantation. In addition to the **Organ Transplant Center,** Memorial's **IVF and Genetics Center** achieved Turkey's first IVF pregnancy via microinjection and is the first fertility center in the nation with an in-house genetics lab for the analysis and resolution of genetic issues prior to fertilization.

Memorial Healthcare Group has established agreements with some of the world's largest insurance firms, including Aetna Global Benefits, AGIS Group, Allianz Worldwide Care, AXA PPP Healthcare, BKK Aktiv, BlueCross BlueShield, Bupa International, Cigna International, Euro-Center, GMC Services International, SOS International (in Denmark, the Netherlands, and the UK), and Vanbreda International. Memorial also has agreements in place for treating elective cases in neurosurgery and orthopedics as well as mammoplasty, otorhinolaryngology, and general, gynecological, and plastic surgery.

Memorial Healthcare Group also operates two medical centers, one on the European side of Istanbul and the other on the Asian side. A new 140-bed general hospital, Atasehir Memorial Hospital, opened in late 2009, and the group has started construction of another new 130-bed complex, Antalya Memorial Hospital, in southern Turkey.

Specialties

✦ Audiology

✦ Cardiology and cardiovascular surgery

✦ Dentistry

✦ Dermatology

✦ Ear, nose, and throat

✦ Emergency medicine

✦ Endocrinology, diabetes, and metabolic disease

✦ Gastroenterology

✦ General surgery

✦ Health checkups

✦ Hepatology

✦ Intensive care

✦ Internal medicine

✦ IVF and pre-fertilization genetic analysis

✦ Medical aesthetics

✦ Neonatology

✦ Nephrology

✦ Neurology and neurosurgery

✦ Nuclear medicine

✦ Obstetrics and gynecology

✦ Ophthalmology

✦ Organ transplantation

✦ Orthopedics, traumatology, and sports medicine

✦ Pediatrics

✦ Physical therapy and rehabilitation

✦ Plastic and reconstructive surgery

✦ Radiology and interventional radiology

✦ Urology (including andrology)

Services Provided for International Patients

✦ Initial screening and diagnosis

✦ Physician evaluation and recommendations

✦ Cost estimates for anticipated treatment

✦ Package pricing that includes all medical, social, and accommodations costs

✦ Appointment scheduling

✦ Accommodations and transportation arrangement for patients and families

✦ Airport pickup and dropoff

✦ Admissions coordination

✦ English-speaking staff and language interpretation

✦ Memorial Guest House services for patients and families

Achievements and Awards

✦ 2002: Turkey's first JCI-accredited hospital

✦ 2002: Turkey's first private hospital to perform endostent applications

✦ 2004: Turkey's first private hospital to carry out differentiation of myocardial cells from embryonic stem cells

✦ 2006: Turkey's first private hospital to perform a blood-type-incompatible pediatric liver transplant

✦ 2008: Turkey's first private hospital to employ yttrium-90 microspheres for treating liver cancer

✦ 2008: Designated one of "52 Best International Hospitals Americans Can Visit" by *U.S. News & World Report*

Feature Story

A Kidney Transplant at Istanbul Memorial Hospital

When Alti Altiyev, a citizen of Turkmenistan, consulted a doctor about a head cold, a more serious problem emerged—Altiyev was suffering from renal failure. For the next ten years, he visited numerous physicians and spent much of his time undergoing dialysis in hospitals. He says, "Though I continued to live, I was just like a dead man. Each day I had was like a nightmare."

At age 32 and married with four children, Altiyev went to a Turkish hospital in Turkmenistan, where the doctors referred him to Istanbul Memorial Hospital. Dr. Burak Kocak, the director of renal transplantation at Memorial's Organ Transplant Center, examined Altiyev and decided that a kidney transplant was urgently needed.

Altiyev's brother-in-law, Annageldi Altinyew, donated a kidney without hesitation. "I know what my brother-in-law has gone through for the last ten years. I once gave him blood, and now I donated him my kidney," Altinyew said. The operation went well, and both men returned healthy to Turkmenistan.

"He had a dramatic change following the transplant. Now he has gone back to his country having regained his health. We hope that he won't need to go to the hospital again except for [followup] examinations," says Dr. Kocak. Altiyev reports, "If I had known that the transplant would be this easy, I would have come to Turkey much earlier for the operation. I lagged behind in many fields, including my job, due to this disease. I could not eat or drink water as I wished. Now, I can eat what I want. I am grateful to my Turkish physicians."

Altiyev's family physician, Dr. Sirmamedov Aleg, hopes that others will follow in his patient's footsteps. "Ten thousand people in Turkmenistan are receiving dialysis treatment for renal failure. Unfortunately, it is not possible to perform an organ transplant in Turkmenistan, and almost nobody knows that this disorder can be treated that easily by means of a renal transplant. A number of people who are aware of the transplant option cannot afford to go abroad and have a transplant. Dialysis machines prove inadequate for those who are treated in hospitals. I hope that patients will be more informed of this issue so nobody will lose his life to renal failure."

Kent Hospital

8229/1 Sok. No. 56
Cigli
Izmir, TURKEY 35580
Tel: 90 232 398.1100
Fax: 90 232 386.7071
Email: info@kenthospital.com
Web: www.internationalkent.com

Kent Hospital was founded in 1999 as one of the largest and most modern hospitals in southeastern Europe. On nearly 9 acres (about 3.6 hectares) of land, the campus was built following American Institute of Architects guidelines and in consultation with the Mayo Clinic in Rochester, Minnesota, on facility design, medical guidelines, and administrative protocols. The hospital is a full-service medical complex offering tertiary-care services in a range of specialties, and it received JCI accreditation in 2006.

With 135 beds, 21 intensive care beds, and six operating theaters, Kent employs 143 full-time physicians, including 60 surgeons, and 450 visiting surgeons. Most of the physicians and a number of additional staff members speak English. Other languages spoken include Arabic, Bulgarian, French, German, Greek, Italian, Russian, and Spanish.

Some of the procedures most frequently performed at Kent include liver and kidney transplantation, coronary angiography and digital subtraction angiography, coronary artery bypass surgery, heart valve replacement, hip and knee replacement, IVF, spinal fusion, stereotaxic surgery, deep brain stimulation, sleep apnea and snoring surgery, head and neck cancer surgery, voice surgery, laser and radical retropubic prostatectomy, percutaneous nephrolithotripsy, and intrauterine fetal diagnosis and treatment, such as ventriculo-amniotic shunting. Kent also offers the full range of minimally invasive and endoscopic surgical procedures, including functional endoscopic surgery, laparoscopic hysterectomy, and laparoscopic-assisted vaginal hysterectomy.

Digitally generated images from bone densitometry, coronary angiography, nuclear medicine, and radiology are made available for use within the hospital and to local and international medical practitioners in a fashion that maintains patient confidentiality. Kent's laboratory is certified for testing all biochemical, hematological, hormonal, and microbiological parameters.

Kent's **Cardiology Diagnostic Unit** is equipped for echocardiography, EKG and Holter monitoring, and EKG stress testing. The unit provides angioplasty, coronary angiography, pacemaker implantation, and stenting. The hospital's specialty centers include the **Diabetes Center, IVF Center, Kidney and**

Liver Transplant Center, Plastic Surgery Center, Sleep Disorder Center, and **Urology Center.**

Kent's package pricing includes

✦ pre-operative consultation

✦ operating room charges (including recovery room, facilities, equipment, and nursing services)

✦ medical equipment and supplies for the procedure (excluding replacement parts)

✦ post-operative in-hospital physiotherapy (as needed)

✦ accommodation in pre- and post-surgical intensive care unit and subsequent private room (as needed)

✦ routine laboratory tests for the procedure as ordered by the attending physician

✦ cardiac EKG investigation and radiology x-ray studies (as needed)

✦ routine medications used during admission and the procedure

✦ doctor fees (surgeon, assistant surgeon, anesthesiologist, physical therapy, and rehabilitation)

✦ roundtrip ground transfers from Izmir's airport

✦ companion's stay at hospital and standard meals

✦ multilanguage translation services

Kent recently opened Alsancak Medical Center, a state-of-the-art multispecialty outpatient clinic, to meet the growing demand of patients in Izmir's city center.

Specialties

+ Aesthetic/cosmetic and plastic surgery
+ Cardiology and cardiovascular surgery
+ Diabetes
+ Emergency medicine
+ Endoscopic and minimally invasive surgery
+ Gastroenterology
+ General surgery
+ Gynecological surgery
+ Internal medicine
+ IVF
+ Neurology and neurosurgery
+ Nuclear medicine
+ Ophthalmology
+ Organ transplantation
+ Orthopedics and traumatology
+ Pediatrics and pediatric surgery
+ Physical therapy and rehabilitation
+ Radiology
+ Urology

Services Provided for International Patients

+ International medical services Web site
+ Appointment scheduling

✦ Flight reservations and confirmations

✦ Accommodations arrangement

✦ Airport pickup and local transportation

✦ Assistance before, during, and after hospitalization

✦ Direct admission

✦ Language interpretation

✦ Medical referrals

✦ Liaison with evaluation agents, employers, and insurance companies

✦ Sightseeing tours

✦ Free use of laptop with Webcam and wireless Internet access

✦ Current editions of international newspapers, magazines, and books, DVD collection of international movies, and satellite television (US, UK, and other European channels)

Achievements and Awards

✦ Patient satisfaction rate of 95 percent

✦ 2006: Aegean region's first hospital to achieve JCI accreditation

✦ 2007: Turkey's first private hospital to perform a pancreas transplant

✦ 2007: Turkey's largest number of kidney transplants among all private hospitals

✦ 2007: Kariyer.net "Value for People" Award

Feature Story

A California Man Undergoes Brain Surgery at Kent Hospital

John and Mary W., a retired couple from California, were very excited about their summer plans. They had booked a cruise months in advance, eager to experience many cultures and relax while visiting idyllic islands and ports around the Mediterranean.

Once they boarded their cruise ship, John and Mary were relaxing, having fun, and enjoying the scenery—until Mary woke one night, surprised and frightened to hear John breathing roughly. He was having an epileptic seizure; he'd never had one before. The ship's doctor began to stabilize John while calling for transport to the closest emergency center. Fortunately, the ship was approaching its next port of call, Kusadasi in Turkey, and as soon as it docked, John was whisked off by an advanced resuscitation ambulance team to Kent Hospital in Izmir, an hour away.

John was evaluated by the emergency medicine specialist on duty, scanned in the nearby radiology department (where MRI and spiral CT are available 24/7), and treated to prevent further seizures. He was diagnosed with a meningioma, a benign brain tumor. Impressed with the efficient and comprehensive care and consultations, John decided to stay in the hospital's intensive care unit for 24 hours of observation and stabilization.

The following day, John and Mary chose to stay at Kent instead of being evacuated to a hospital near their home in California. One of Kent's in-house neurosurgeons, a professor with training in the US and more than 20 years of experience, then took John to the operating room. The surgeon and his support staff performed a craniotomy and successfully removed the tumor completely. After an additional day of monitoring in intensive care, John was transferred to a single-patient room with an extra bed for Mary, where he recovered well and without complications. He and his wife stayed connected with their family through Kent's free laptop computer and wireless Internet service.

John and Mary were pleased not only with the excellent and up-to-date treatment he received, but also with its low cost—a fraction of what it would have cost in the US. After returning home, John continued to enjoy retired life, and Mary wrote an article for her local newspaper describing the hospitality of the Turkish people and the high standards of medical care that John had received at Kent.

MESA Hospital

Yasam Cad. No. 5
Sogutozu
Ankara, TURKEY 06510
Tel: 90 312 292.9900
Fax: 90 312 292.9910
Email: info@mesahastanesi.com.tr
Web: www.mesahastanesi.com.tr

MESA Hospital opened its doors in 2004 and earned its JCI accreditation two years later. Most of the hospital's 100 physicians and surgeons and 86 full-time staff members speak English; other languages spoken include Arabic, French, German, and Russian. This 100-bed facility is best known for cardiology and cardiovascular surgery, cataract surgery, colorectal surgery, neurosurgery (including spinal surgery and procedures for epilepsy and Parkinson's disease), and orthopedics. The procedures most frequently performed at MESA are cataract removal, coronary angioplasty, and spinal surgery. The hospital treats 1,500 international patients annually, some 800 of them from the US and Canada.

MESA is also known for its obstetric services, as the hospital is a center for labor and delivery among pregnant women visiting the area (120 in 2008), roughly a third of them affiliated with the US Air Force Base at Incirlik. The women are invited to MESA about two weeks before their due dates, where they receive a guided tour of the labor and delivery facilities with the hospital's **International Patient's Service Coordinator.** Their registration and paperwork are completed in advance, so everything is ready when the baby arrives.

MESA's specialty centers include the **Center for Spine and Spinal Cord Disorders, Center for Surgery of Liver-Gallbladder-Pancreas, Center for Surgery of Parkinson's Disease, Colorectal Clinic,** and **Dental Clinic.**

Specialties

✦ Anesthesiology

✦ Cardiology and cardiovascular surgery

✦ Dentistry

✦ Dermatology

✦ Ear, nose, and throat

✦ Emergency medicine

✦ Endocrinology and metabolic disease

✦ Gastroenterology

✦ General surgery

+ Internal medicine

+ Neurology and neurosurgery

+ Obstetrics and gynecology

+ Ophthalmology

+ Orthopedics and traumatology

+ Pediatrics

+ Physical therapy and rehabilitation

+ Plastic and reconstructive surgery

+ Respiratory medicine

+ Urology

Services Provided for International Patients

+ Consultation on treatment plans

+ Appointment scheduling

+ Travel and transportation coordination

+ Accomodations arrangement

+ Language interpretation and translation of medical reports

+ Assistance with medical insurance

+ Treatment followup

+ Seminars (maternal services and infant care, diabetes management, glaucoma treatment and cataract surgery, and skin care and choice of cosmetics)

+ Arrangements for special services, tours, religious and cultural activities, sightseeing, sports, and recreation

Feature Story

International Patients Give Birth at MESA Hospital

Pregnant women from overseas are nothing new in the Obstetrics and Gynecology Department at MESA Hospital. According to the hospital's managing director, Metin Atak, MESA is receiving more and more Canadian and American women every year, along with ever-growing numbers of other international patients. Canadian citizen Kimberly Bewick, who recently gave birth to her second child at MESA, says she chose this hospital for several reasons. "Being able to give birth in my own room inspired me," she reports. "Furthermore, the nurses' and medical staff's constant care and attention made me feel very safe. And my family in Canada even attended the delivery online."

Yeditepe University Hospital

Devlet Yolu
Ankara Cad. No. 102–104
Kozyatagi
Istanbul, TURKEY 34752
Tel: 90 216 578.4000
Fax: 90 216 469.3796
Email: internationalpatients@yeditepe.edu.tr
Web: www.yeditepehealthcare.com

Yeditepe University Hospital opened in 2005 and received JCI accreditation in 2007. This 170-bed hospital serves about 1,000 international patients annually. Its facilities include eight operating rooms, a general intensive care unit, and specialized intensive care units for newborns as well as cardiovascular surgery, neurosurgery, and coronary patients. Yeditepe employs more than 150 physicians and surgeons and more than 800 additional full-time staff members, and maintains international academic collaborations in the US with the Cleveland Clinic (Ohio), the M.D. Anderson Cancer Center (Houston), and Memorial Sloan-Kettering Cancer Center (New York).

Among Yeditepe's specialty clinics are the **Organ Transplant Center, Clinic for Breast Diseases, Clinic for Cerebrovascular Diseases, Clinic for Diagnosis and Treatment of Lung Cancer, Clinic for Epilepsy, Clinic for Health-Risk Evaluation, Clinic for Microsurgery, Clinic for Sexual Dysfunctions, Clinic for Sleeping Disorders, Clinic for Smoking Cessation,** and **Diabetic Foot Clinic.**

Yeditepe's centers of excellence include

✦ **Cardiovascular and Thoracic Surgery Department,** offering a wide range of treatments, including heart failure surgery as well as diagnosis and comprehensive treatment of lung cancer. Major airway surgery is another field of expertise.

✦ **Ear-Nose-Throat Clinic,** where hearing and voice are primary interests. Treatment modalities include cochlear implantation, hearing aids, laryngoplastic surgery, and phonomicrosurgery. The clinic's physicians have expertise in communicative disorders and the performing arts.

✦ **Genetics Center,** where researchers are evaluating the use of gene therapy in the treatment of malignant tumors and for the prevention of adverse effects associated with organ transplantation.

✦ **Imaging Center,** employing angiography, digital mammography, Gamma Camera, 3-Tesla MRI, multislice CT, and PET-CT (to detect cancerous cells). In 2008 Yeditepe became a clinical research center for the development of 3-Tesla MRI technologies through a partnership agreement with Philips Electronics.

✦ **Infertility Center,** utilizing a wide variety of assisted reproduction technologies to provide the full range of assessment, treatment, and followup services.

✦ **Neurological Sciences Center,** where multidisciplinary teams of specialists conduct studies in brain and vascular surgery, epilepsy, neuro-oncology, spinal surgery, and trauma, as well as functional, pediatric, peripheral, and stereotactic neurosurgery. Cortical mapping and intraoperative monitoring of evoked potentials and cranial nerve EMG are employed in the support of highly sophisticated brain surgeries.

✦ **Orthopedics and Traumatology Department,** offering 24-hour microsurgery to repair fine vessel and nerve injuries with the use of operative microscopes. Vertebral fractures, infections, tumors, and congenital or acquired curvatures are successfully treated with modern surgical techniques.

✦ **Plastic and Reconstructive Surgery Department,** providing a wide range of treatments that includes correction of congenital malformations (cleft lip and palate, craniofacial irregularity, ear deformity, vascular tumors, and anomalies of the breast, genitalia, and hand); reconstructive surgery (breast reconstruction, emergency and elective reconstruction of maxillofacial trauma, facial reanimation and reconstruction, treatment of burn complications, and scar revision); excision of head and neck tumors, parotid tumors, and malignant and benign soft-tissue tumors; and the full range of cosmetic procedures, from tummy tuck to facial rejuvenation via fat cell transfer.

✦ **Stem Cell Transplantation Unit,** diagnosing and treating malignant and nonmalignant hematological disease as well as solid tumors. Autologous and allogeneic bone marrow transplants are performed. The unit is supported by the hospital's **Extracorporeal Photopheresis Unit** in treating T-cell lymphoma and related disorders.

✦ **Urology Department,** successfully performing minimally invasive surgery with imaging techniques that allow visualization of the operative field at 10–20× magnification. Surgery performed in this way is more precise, and blood loss is minimized.

Yeditepe University also includes a fully equipped **Dental Hospital. Yeditepe University Eye Center** opened in 2007 and offers cataract surgery, corneal disease and glaucoma treatment, oculoplastic surgery, pediatric ophthalmology, and refractive surgery, using the latest in laser technology. The facility has 15 examination rooms and four operating rooms. It employs 13 physicians and surgeons who speak English, French, and German.

Specialties

✦ Breast disease

✦ Cardiology and cardiovascular surgery

✦ Cerebrovascular disease

✦ Diabetes

✦ Ear, nose, and throat

✦ Endocrinology and metabolic disease

✦ Gastroenterology

✦ General surgery

✦ Genetics

✦ Health checkups

✦ Hematology

✦ IVF

✦ Microsurgery

✦ Nephrology

✦ Neurology and neurosurgery

✦ Nuclear medicine

✦ Obstetrics and gynecology

✦ Oncology

✦ Ophthalmology (adult and pediatric)

✦ Organ transplantation

✦ Orthopedics and traumatology

✦ Pathology

✢ Pediatrics and pediatric surgery

✢ Plastic and reconstructive surgery

✢ Rheumatology

✢ Speech-language pathology, cochlear implantation, and vocal surgery

✢ Stem cell (bone marrow) transplantation

✢ Thoracic surgery

✢ Urology

Services Provided for International Patients

✢ International medical services Web site

✢ Consultation prior to arrival

✢ Telemedicine for second opinion and full electronic medical record capability

✢ Appointment scheduling

✢ Flight reservation and confirmation

✢ Accommodations arrangement

✢ Airport pickup and local transportation

✢ Assistance before, during, and after hospitalization

✢ Direct admission

✢ Language interpretation

✢ Sightseeing tours

✢ Medical information exchange with home-country health-care providers

✦ Communication with international insurance companies

✦ Respectful approach to religious and cultural preferences

Achievements and Awards

✦ 2005: Turkey's first (and only) private university hospital blood bank licensed by the Ministry of Health

✦ 2006: Turkey's first double-balloon small-bowel endoscopy

✦ 2006: Turkey's first permanent artificial heart pump surgery

✦ 2006: World's first window anterior commissure relaxation laryngoplasty (a type of voice surgery)

✦ 2007: World's first free vascularized fibula grafting for extensive knee osteonecrosis

✦ 2007–2010: Turkey's first (and only) Artificial Heart Pump Project

✦ 2008: Turkey's first implantable miniature left-ventricle-assisted (Impella) coronary artery surgery

✦ 2008: Santez Project (drug-releasing biodegradable polymer cardiac stent)

✦ 2008: Turkey's first National Cochlear Implant Project

Feature Story

A Canadian Chooses Cosmetic Surgery at Yeditepe University Hospital

Carine, a 54-year-old university lecturer from Canada, wanted antiaging cosmetic surgery. Looking for the best procedures, doctors, and hospitals in Istanbul, she did considerable research among people she knew and online—and discovered Yeditepe University Hospital through the English version of *Yeditepe Health Magazine*. After consulting with four other doctors, she selected a surgical team at Yeditepe.

"I chose Yeditepe because its international reputation and standards are very high, especially the plastic surgery team. Compared to all other doctors I consulted, Yeditepe surgeons possess all the qualities I had hoped for and more. From my first consultation onward, my confidence increased with every meeting. I was offered the most intelligent, the most progressive, and least-invasive solutions. My doctor is an artist at heart. He has an extraordinarily kind, gentle, patient, considerate, and generous manner," says Carine.

She underwent facial rejuvenation with fat cell transfer, a same-day surgical procedure performed under local anesthesia. After the operation, she reports having experienced very little pain and no complications.

"This hospital is obviously world-class," Carine says. "My pre-operative care was thorough and excellent, my private room with a view of the Bosphorus was amazing, and my hours of surgery were painless and stress-free. A lovely nurse sat and read to me in English. Even my check-out was easy and efficient."

Other JCI-Accredited Hospitals

Turkey has more JCI-accredited hospitals than any other country in the world. The previous section featured 11 hospitals and hospital groups—most of them JCI-accredited—that are actively seeking international patients. They are not, however, the only facilities serving medical travelers in Turkey. You may wish to contact one of the other JCI-accredited hospitals listed below.

Alman Hastanesi (German Hospital)

Siraselviler Cad. No. 119
Taksim
Istanbul, TURKEY 80060
Tel: 90 212 293.2150
Fax: 90 212 293.4752; 90 212 252.3911
Email: almanhastanesi@uhg.com.tr
Web: http://almanhastanesi.com.tr/genel.htm

Dunya Eye Hospital (World Eye Centers)

Nispetiye Cad.
Yanarsu Sok. No. 1
Etiler
Istanbul, TURKEY 34337
Tel: 90 212 444.4469; 90 212 362.3232
Fax: 90 212 257.0924
Email: dunyagoz@dunyagoz.com
Web: www.worldeyelasik.com

Ege Saglik Hospital

1399 Sok. No. 25
Alsancak
Izmir, TURKEY 35220
Tel: 90 232 463.7700
Fax: 90 232 463.0371
Email: msucuoglu@egesaglik.com.tr
Web: www.egesaglik.com.tr

Hacettepe University Adult Hospital

Hacettepe University Hospitals
Sihhiye
Ankara, TURKEY 06100
Tel: 90 312 305.1101
Fax: 90 312 311.0994
Email: tkutluk@hacettepe.edu.tr
Web: www.hacettepe.com.tr

Medical Park Antalya Hospital

Fener Mah.
Tekelioglu Cad. No. 7
Lara
Antalya, TURKEY 07230
Tel: 90 242 314.3434
Fax: 90 242 314.3030
Email: antalya@medicalpark.com.tr
Web: www.medicalpark.com.tr

Medical Park Bahcelievler Hospital

E5 Uzeri, Bahcelievler Metro Station
Yani
Istanbul, TURKEY 34160
Tel: 90 212 484.1484
Fax: 90 212 484.1064
Email: bahcelievler@medicalpark.com.tr
Web: www.medicalpark.com.tr

Medical Park Bursa Hospital

Hasim Iscan Cad.
Fomara Meydani No. 1
Osmangazi
Bursa, TURKEY 16050
Tel: 90 224 270.6000
Fax: 90 224 224.8635
Email: bursa@medicalpark.com.tr
Web: www.medicalpark.com.tr

Medical Park Goztepe Hospital

E5 Uzeri
Goztepe Kavsagi
Goztepe, Kadikoy
Istanbul, TURKEY 34732
Tel: 90 216 468.4444
Fax: 90 216 468.4567
Email: goztepe@medicalpark.com.tr
Web: www.medicalpark.com.tr

Medicana Bahcelievler Hospital

Eski Londra Asfalti No. 2
Bahcelievler
Istanbul, TURKEY 34180
Tel: 90 212 449.1449
Fax: 90 212 556.1913
Email: info@medicana.com.tr
Web: www.medicana.com.tr

Medicana Camlica Hospital

Alemdag Cad. No. 85
Uskudar
Istanbul, TURKEY 34767
Tel: 90 216 521.3030
Fax: 90 216 335.8636
Email: info@medicana.com.tr
Web: www.medicana.com.tr

Sema Hospital

Yali Mah.
Sahil Yolu Sok. No. 16
Dragos, Maltepe
Istanbul, TURKEY 34844
Tel: 90 216 444.7362
Fax: 90 216 352.8359
Email: sema@semasaglik.com
Web: www.semahastanesi.com.tr

TDV Ozel 29 Mayis Hastanesi

Aydinlar Mah.
Dikmen Cad. No. 312
Cankaya
Ankara, TURKEY
Tel: 90 312 593.2929
Fax: 90 312 593.2998
Email: halklailiskiler.ankara@29mayis.com.tr
Web: www.29mayis.com.tr

Uludag University School of Health Services

Gorukle Campus
Bursa, TURKEY 16059
Tel: 90 224 295.0000
Fax: 90 224 295.0019
Email: suam@uludag.edu.tr
Web: http://tip.uludag.edu.tr

Vehbi Koc Foundation American Hospital

Azizbey Sok. No. 1
Nakkastepe, Kuzguncuk
Istanbul, TURKEY
Tel: 90 212 444.3777
Email: info@vkv.org.tr
Web: www.vkv.org.tr

Health Travel Agents
Serving Turkey

BridgeHealth International, Inc.

5299 Denver Tech Center Blvd., Ste. 800
Greenwood Village, CO 80111
Tel: 800 680.1366 (US and Canada toll-free); 303 457.5734
Fax: 303 779.0366
Email: info@bridgehealthintl.com
Web: www.bridgehealthintl.com

BridgeHealth International (BHI) sends patients to Costa Rica, India, Mexico, Singapore, Thailand, Turkey, and other countries. Serving the business and insurance markets as well as individual consumers, the BHI staff have a lot of experience in steering clients through the medical travel process.

Before accepting a client, BHI screens for health and "travelability." Clients pay no facilitation fees; the fees are paid by the agency's list of approved physicians, clinics, and hospitals (JCI-accredited or equivalent only). Services include passport and visa assistance, airline reservations, medical consultations, medical records transfer assistance, full in-country concierge services, pre-operative and post-operative counseling, and followup care arrangements. BHI coordinates a full range of care from bariatric, cosmetic, dental, and stem cell procedures to cardiovascular surgery, neurosurgery, organ transplantation, and orthopedic surgery.

Companion Global Healthcare, Inc.

c/o BlueCross BlueShield of South Carolina
I-20 at Alpine Rd., AX-724
Columbia, SC 29219
Tel: 800 906.7065 (US toll-free)
Fax: 803 264.7063
Email: info@companionglobalhealthcare.com
Web: www.companionglobalhealthcare.com

Companion Global Healthcare started out working with hospitals in Ireland and Thailand, and it has since expanded its reach to include Brazil, Costa Rica, Germany, India, Mexico, Singapore, South Korea, Taiwan, and Turkey. Although this agency is a wholly owned subsidiary of BlueCross BlueShield of South Carolina, anyone in the US can use its services. At present, followup care upon return from medical travel is provided in South Carolina only, but that situation may change as Companion Global works with BlueCross BlueShield and other insurance carriers to expand their activities and support of low-cost, fully credentialed medical travel.

Companion Global's call center offers help to health travelers in a whopping 20 languages! The agency's standard package includes case management, medical record transfer, and travel coordination. Depending on the patient's diagnosis, treatment, and benefit plan, insurance carriers are paying significant portions of the cost. Uninsured customers and clients of other insurance companies pay overseas providers directly. Companion Global estimates savings on procedures such as total hip replacement at 40–85 percent below US prices.

GUSIB

Dr. Kazim Lakay Sok.
Adil Ozev Apt. No. 8/7
Fenerbahce
Istanbul, TURKEY 34726
Tel: 90 216 355.1755
Fax: 90 216 355.1755
Email: info@gusib.com
Web: www.gusib.com

Serving medical travelers since 2002, this Istanbul-based agency arranges travel to and from Austria, Germany, the Netherlands, Turkey, and the UK. The agency has assisted nearly 400 patients since 2004 and is now serving a steady stream of about ten per month. Staff members speak English and German.

GUSIB allows patients to contact physicians and treatment centers directly. Its standard package includes flights, transportation to and from the airport, hotel, transfers, some guided tours, and hospital arrangements. Package pricing is available for certain procedures; for example, the laser eye-treatment package costs about 1,500 euros (approximately US$2,050) for patients from European countries.

Heal in Turkey

Divan Yolu Cad.
Bicki Yurdu Sok. No. 12/A
Sultanahmet
Istanbul, TURKEY 34400
Tel: 90 212 511.8600
Fax: 90 212 512.5606
Email: info@healinturkey.com
Web: www.healinturkey.com

Heal in Turkey has been in business since 1999, arranging health travel for patients from France, Germany, Hungary, North Cyprus, Russia, Switzerland, and the UK. The agency currently serves about 100 medical travelers annually.

Heal in Turkey's standard services include travel arrangements, airport transfers, a 24-hour hotline, case management, medical consulting, and treatment arrangements; examination by the medical team (surgeon, anesthetist, doctor, etc.) before and after treatment, all routine checkups before surgery (blood work, EKG, etc.), all medications, and extra prostheses (as needed before, during, and after surgery); hospital stay and meals for a companion; and visits and orientation at the hospital and at the hotel area after hospital discharge. Extra fees may be incurred for hotel rooms, private sightseeing tours, and intensive care.

Heal in Turkey offers package prices for bariatric surgery, cosmetic surgery, dentistry, and laser eye treatments. Custom packages can be arranged for health checkup screening, hair transplant, heart surgery, infertility and sterility treatment, orthopedic surgery, various diagnostic and treatment procedures (such as angioplasty), radiological diagnostic procedures (such as CT scans), and urological and anthological procedures (such as sexual health surgery). Also popular are spa holidays and trips to thermal resorts. Heal in Turkey's clients often recover at the History Hotel in Istanbul.

Healthbase Online, Inc.

287 Auburn St.
Newton, MA 02466
Tel: 888 691.4584 (US and Canada toll-free); 617 418.3436
Fax: 800 986.9230 (US and Canada toll-free)
Email: info.hb@healthbase.com
Web: www.healthbase.com

Healthbase Online, a Boston-based medical tourism facilitator, is organized as a one-stop source for medical travel logistics and concierge services. Healthbase connects patients with internationally accredited (mainly JCI-accredited) hospitals in Belgium, Brazil, Costa Rica, Hungary, India, Malaysia, Mexico, New Zealand, Panama, the Philippines, Singapore, South Korea, Spain, Thailand, Turkey, and the US. The agency expects soon to expand its services to Argentina, Australia, Canada, the Czech Republic, El Salvador, Guatemala, Jordan, Poland, South Africa, Taiwan, and the UK.

Healthbase prides itself on exclusive, friendly, and personalized care and round-the-clock customer support. Promising cost savings to organizations and reduced healthcare premiums for clients, the agency serves individual consumers, self-funded businesses, insurers, benefits plan consultants, third-party administrators, and users of consumer-directed healthcare plans or voluntary benefit plans. Healthbase offers customized corporate medical tourism plans for employers and insurance companies. Other services include medical and dental loan financing and travel insurance.

Through the Healthbase online research tool—designated "Best Website for Accessing International Medical Information for Patients/Consumers" in 2007 by *Consumer Health World*—members can explore the medical procedures available and the hospitals offering them, correspond with hospitals and physicians, and share digitized medical records. This secure Web-based system provides instant connectivity with the agency's partner hospitals for speedy, efficient, and effective handling of medical travel inquiries.

ICEPWORLD

81 Oxford St.
London, UNITED KINGDOM W1D 2EU
Tel: 44 20 7580.3106
Email: london@sanatoliacare.com
Web: www.sanatoliacare.com

ICEPWORLD has been operating since 2005, sending four or five patients each month to hospitals in Turkey. The agency allows patients to contact physicians and treatment centers directly. Its packages include accommodations, transportation to and from the airport, ambulance services, and excursions.

Mediline Worldwide Health Tourism

Ahi Evren Cad. Ata Center No. 1
Kat. 5, Maslak
Istanbul, TURKEY 34398
Tel: 90 212 276.1131
Fax: 90 212 276.1132
Email: info@medilineeurope.com
Web: www.medilineeurope.com

This agency, established in 2006, serves about 20 patients each month, most of them from Bulgaria, Georgia, Romania, and Ukraine. The majority undergo LASIK eye surgery in Istanbul. Mediline Worldwide Health Tourism staff members speak Bulgarian, English, Romanian, and Russian, and they can arrange for translators in nearly all languages. The agency arranges video conferences between patient and physician. Hoping to attract more patients from the US and Canada, Mediline's "Guardian Service" promises a bilingual native English speaker to correspond with patients before they leave home, receive them at the airport, escort them to doctor's appointments, and support patients and their families during the procedure and hospital stay. The most frequently used hospitals are Acibadem Healthcare Group and Anadolu Medical Center.

Med Journeys

120 South Mountain Ave.
Montclair, NJ 07042
Tel: 888 633.5769 (US toll-free); 212 931.0557
Fax: 212 656.1134
Email: mj-info@medjourneys.com
Web: www.medjourneys.com

This agency sends most of its clients to Costa Rica, India, Mexico, and Thailand, but has also cemented relationships with hospitals in other countries, including Turkey. Since its establishment in 2005, Med Journeys has sent more than 350 patients abroad, and the numbers are growing.

Med Journeys' standard package includes the medical procedure, accommodations during recuperation (including three meals daily), airfare, private transportation in the host country, and premium concierge services. Extra fees are generally charged for optional tours, companions, extended stays, and added medical procedures. Med Journeys encourages clients to contact physicians directly to check references and ask questions about procedures and treatments.

MedRetreat

2042 Laurel Valley Dr.
Vernon Hills, IL 60061
Tel: 877 876.3373 (US toll-free); 443 451.9996
Fax: 847 680.0484
Email: customerservice@medretreat.com
Web: www.medretreat.com

In operation since 2003, MedRetreat is one of the better-established US-based health travel agencies, sending patients to Brazil, Costa Rica, El Salvador, India, Malaysia, Mexico, South Africa, Thailand, and Turkey. Members receive personalized service through a boutique-style program designed to meet their specific needs. This process includes acquiring hospital information, physicians' credentials, and doctors' consultations; collecting and disseminating medical records; completing price quotations; and arranging procedures, passport and visa acquisition, air travel, travel insurance, financing, destination ground transportation, post-operative hotel booking, and more.

MedRetreat provides 24-hour access to a US program manager, concierge services in the treatment destination, communications while abroad, and assistance once back home. MedRetreat also offers an unconditional money-back guarantee. Its services are free on a first-come, first-served basis.

Patients Without Borders

304 Newbury St. #364
Boston, MA 02115
Tel: 617 708.4229
Fax: 617 648.4426
Email: jeff.carter@patientswithoutborders.us
Web: www.patientswithoutborders.us

Patients Without Borders, established in 2008, is gaining experience in serving medical travelers to Turkey as well as Argentina, Costa Rica, Malaysia, the Philippines, Singapore, South Korea, Taiwan, and the US.

Standard packages include transfer of medical records, air travel arrangements, airport pickup and dropoff, transportation to and from medical appointments, pre-operative visits in the host country, operative costs (including hospital room, operating room, anesthesia, anesthesiologist, surgeon, and associated fees), post-operative visits, and planning for aftercare back home (including identifying an aftercare provider). Additional charges may be incurred for personal telephone services, special Internet services, meals and room for a companion, sightseeing tours, nonmedical transportation, and extra medical services.

This agency promises to work closely with its clients' at-home and host-country physicians to ensure continuity of care. Patients Without Borders also works with insurance companies to determine whether an overseas procedure can be covered.

Patients Without Borders is not affiliated in any way with *Patients Beyond Borders.*™

Planet Hospital

23679 Calabasas Rd., Ste. 150
Calabasas, CA 91302
Tel: 800 243.0172 (US toll-free); 818 591.1668
Fax: 818 665.4801
Email: rudy@planethospital.com
Web: www.planethospital.com

Rudy Rupak founded Planet Hospital in 2002, after being impressed with the quality of care his fiancée received when she fell ill in Thailand, and the agency has since sent more than 3,000 patients abroad for medical care. It currently serves 14 countries: Belgium, Costa Rica, Cyprus, El Salvador, India, Malaysia, Malta, Mexico, Panama, the Philippines, Singapore, South Korea, Thailand, and Turkey. Planet Hospital's in-country concierges take care of clients from the moment they land to the moment they leave, and its representatives personally inspect every hospital and doctor the agency recommends.

Planet Hospital currently works with several self-insured employers who have contracted its services to help their employees save money. Specialties include cardiovascular procedures, cosmetic surgery, dentistry, fertility/reproduction (including surrogacy), oncology, and orthopedics. Planet Hospital is the only medical travel agency that has been a member of the Better Business Bureau since 2002 with an AA rating.

The agency's Web site offers a comprehensive list of major hospitals in its service areas, along with a sampling of its top recommended physicians. A robust testimonials page features real clients with real names. At this writing, Planet Hospital is sending five patients per day abroad for treatment from its offices in California, Canada, France, Saudi Arabia, and the UK.

Satori World Medical

591 Camino De La Reina, Ste. 407
San Diego, CA 92108
Tel: 619 704.2000
Fax: 619 704.2049
Email: j.yarbrough@satoriworldmedical.com
Web: www.satoriworldmedical.com

Satori World Medical started operating in 2007, and its growing network includes hospitals in Costa Rica, India, Mexico, the Philippines, Singapore, Thailand, and Turkey. Satori's patient advocates are nurses who coordinate all inquiries, from discussing procedures with the patient and facilitating medical records transfer to scheduling followup care and educating companions on their responsibilities. The agency's travel care coordinators schedule procedure dates with the hospital, make airline and hotel reservations, coordinate ground transportation, and provide 24-hour customer service. Package pricing includes all procedure, hospital, and physician fees; roundtrip airfare for the patient and a companion; a two-week stay at an Intercontinental hotel; and a personal accident insurance policy.

VisitandCare.com

Cigdem Sok. No. 7
Coskuncan Apt. D:1
Florya
Istanbul, TURKEY 34153
Tel: 90 212 573.0221
Fax: 90 212 573.8909
Email: contact@visitandcare.com
Web: www.visitandcare.com

Established in 2007, VisitandCare.com is one of the first medical travel agencies in Turkey to serve patients from all over the globe. It currently works with more than 50 hospitals in 22 countries. VisitandCare.com does not charge patients for its services, as the agency's fees are covered by its associated hospitals and clinics.

WorldMed Assist

1230 Mountain Side Ct.
Concord, CA 94521
Tel: 866 999.3848 (US toll-free)
Fax: 925 905.5898
Email: info@worldmedassist.com
Web: www.worldmedassist.com

Since opening in 2006, WorldMed Assist has established partnerships with several hospitals and is the medical logistics provider for clients of Swiss Re's Commercial Insurance. The agency aims to provide the highest possible level of customer service, with case management provided by registered nurses, not salespeople. Staff members speak English, Spanish, and

Dutch. WorldMed advertises its highly competitive rates with no markups on surgeries, and it conducts negotiations on the client's behalf with its ongoing partners. The agency and its clients have been featured on BBC, ABC News, Fox News, and NPR's *All Things Considered*.

Turkey: A Nation to See and Love

International travel can be a life-changing experience, and medical travelers can bring back more from their trip than improved health—they can return with an appreciation for a landscape, a culture, and a way of life very different from their own. In Turkey, international patients and their companions can take advantage of the opportunity to sample the sights, sounds, and flavors of urban Istanbul, the historic ruins at Ephesus, or the seaside splendors of Marmaris and Fethiye.

Part Three provides important details to help you plan your medical journey to Turkey—along with some ideas for enjoying the country's unique sights and experiences while you're there.

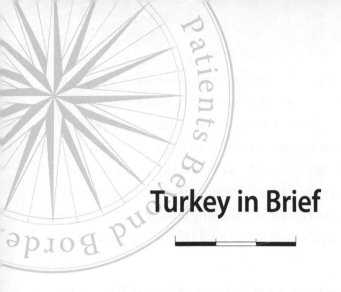

Turkey in Brief

Geography and Climate

Turkey—officially the Republic of Turkey—is strategically posi-tioned at the crossroads of Europe, Asia, and the Middle East. Turkey encompasses the Anatolian peninsula of western Asia, the East Thrace region of Europe, and some islands of the Mar-mara and Aegean seas. Turkey shares its borders with eight other countries: Bulgaria, Greece, Georgia, Armenia, Azerbaijan, Iran, Iraq, and Syria. Its coastline runs about 5,000 miles (about 8,050 kilometers) along the Mediterranean, the Aegean, and the Black seas. The Sea of Marmara and the Turkish Straits—the Bos-phorus and the Dardanelles—separate the European and Asian parts of Turkey.

With a total area of about 301,000 square miles (about 780,580 square kilometers), Turkey is slightly larger than the US state of Texas and larger than France and the UK combined. The landscape varies widely—from coastal plains to mountain pastures, from cedar forests to sweeping steppes. It is home to more than 10,000 species of plants, 3,000 of them endemic to Turkey.

Turkey's climate ranges widely as well. The Southeast is dry, while the Black Sea area is often clothed in mist. The Mediterranean and Aegean areas have mild winters, but the mountainous eastern region experiences months of snow and severe cold. Generally, Turkey's summers are long, warm, and rainless.

Political System and International Relations

Among more than 50 countries with predominantly Muslim populations, Turkey is the only secular democracy. Turkey's modern political system evolved post–World War I under the leadership of Mustafa Kemal Ataturk. A hero of the Turkish national liberation struggle in 1919, Ataturk led his nation to independence and created the Republic of Turkey in 1923. Serving as its president until his death in 1938, he introduced numerous political, social, legal, economic, and cultural reforms that set Turkey on the road to becoming the developed and internationally influential nation it is today.

Turkey has been a multiparty parliamentary democracy since 1947, with legislative power vested in the 550-member Turkish Grand National Assembly, whose members are elected to five-year terms by the votes of all citizens over the age of 18. Turkish women gained the right to vote in 1934, well ahead of women in many other European countries.

Turkey holds memberships in the Council of Europe, North Atlantic Treaty Organization (NATO), Organization for Economic Cooperation and Development (OECD), Organization for Security and Cooperation in Europe, and the G-20, comprising 19 of the world's largest economies plus the European Union (EU). Having become an associate member of the European Economic Community in 1963 and a full member of the EU Customs Union in 1996, Turkey began negotiations for full EU membership in 2005.

The people of Turkey in modern times offer to the world the same sentiment President Ataturk expressed so well in 1933: "I look to the world with an open heart full of pure feelings and friendship."

Economy

Turkey's developed market economy has a rich history of private enterprise. With a gross domestic product (GDP) of nearly US$800 billion and a purchasing power parity per capita of US$9,333, it ranks seventeenth among the world's more than 190 national economies. Annual GDP growth has averaged nearly 7 percent since 2002, and the Istanbul Stock Exchange index has tripled. The US has identified Turkey as one of its ten largest emerging markets. Turkey is Europe's seventh largest trading partner, while Europe is Turkey's main partner and accounts for about half its trade.

Turkey has enjoyed a capitalist boom since 2001. Thanks to a strong entrepreneurial spirit and a highly skilled, cost-effective labor force, Turkish exports exceeded US$107 billion in 2007. A large and expanding domestic market consumed US$170 billion in imports that same year. In recent years, Turkey's market reforms, strong growth, and economic and political stability have attracted ever-growing foreign direct investment, which reached US$22 billion in 2007. The existence of more than 13,900 foreign capital firms ensures a stable and reliable investment environment in Turkey.

The nation's financial sector is well developed in both technology and legal procedures. Turkish finance is built upon a universal banking system and related services, such as insurance, leasing, factoring, and stock brokerage. Turkey offers a competitive tax system. Due to the liberal and secure investment environment, major multinationals are key players in Turkey's economy, and an increasing number of global companies are relocating their Eurasian business units to Istanbul. General Electric, Hewlett-Packard, Johnson & Johnson, Kraft, Microsoft, Pfizer, Procter & Gamble, Toyota, and 3M are a sampling of the leading global corporations operating in Turkey.

Tourism

Turkey's efficient and dynamic tourist industry springs from the country's great diversity of historical treasures, cultural heritage, and natural attractions. Its renowned cuisine, restaurants, bars, entertainment, and cultural activities appeal to tourists from all over the world. Turkey is also a growing destination for trekkers, with the grandest of its snowcapped mountains being the lofty 17,725-foot (5,402-meter) summit of Mount Ararat. And it is a country of rivers, as both the Tigris and Euphrates rise in Turkey.

In 2007 almost 12 million Europeans and 650,000 US citizens enjoyed Turkey's resorts—dubbed the Turkish Riviera—as well as its bustling and historic cities and unique World Heritage Sites, which include the rock-carved dwellings of Cappadocia, the ancient spa-city of Hierapolis atop the hot springs of Pamukkale, and the archaeological site of Troy. A total of 23.3 million people visited Turkey in 2007, and in 2008 the annual total reached nearly 31 million. Turkey is now Europe's leading tourism destination.

Over the last two decades, Turkey has made considerable investments in its infrastructure. In addition to the international airports servicing the main cities and resort destinations, Turkish Airlines offers domestic flights to all major cities and tourist centers. The nation's advanced communication systems network meets the needs of Turkish citizens and international travelers alike.

The accommodations industry offers facilities ranging from supermodern deluxe hotels and holiday complexes to value-priced boutique hotels. Although city hotels, summer resorts, and holiday complexes are the main types of lodging available, numerous winter resorts and spa hotels also operate in many parts of the country. Turkey's top-quality, huge-capacity convention centers feature high-tech equipment and frequently host important gatherings. Smaller meetings are also common, as most high-grade hotels also offer facilities for special events, meetings, and conventions.

Turkey's World-Famous Cuisine

It is said that the world's three major cuisines are Chinese, French, and Turkish. Fully justifying its reputation, Turkish cuisine is always a pleasant surprise for the visitor. With the variety and simplicity of its recipes and the quality of its ingredients, delicious meals are guaranteed!

- Soups are generally based on meat stock and served at the start of the meal. Lentil soup is the most common and best-loved variety.

- *Mezes* are appetizers, often served in great abundance and variety. Examples include fried eggplant (aubergine) with yogurt, *lakerda* (bonito preserved in brine), *pastirma* (pressed beef), fish croquettes, and *cacik* (yogurt and cucumbers). Don't forget to try the spicy meat dumplings called *manti*—but visitors are advised to consume *mezes* sparingly, because there's a great deal more to come.

- Lamb is the basic meat of any Turkish kitchen. Kebabs are plain or marinated meat either stewed or grilled. Pieces of lamb threaded on a skewer and grilled over charcoal are *sis kebab*. *Doner kebab* is a roll of lamb on a vertical skewer rotated parallel to a vertical grill.

- Eggplant is used in a variety of dishes, including eggplant salad and stuffed eggplant. Cooked with onions, garlic, and tomatoes, it is served cold as *imam bayildi*.

- A delicious Turkish specialty is the rice dish *pilav*, which is difficult for the inexperienced cook to prepare. Cooks in the Black Sea region prepare a rice-and-fish variation called *hamsili pilav*. Another interesting specialty from that region is *miroloto*, a bread containing cabbage, chard, and onions.

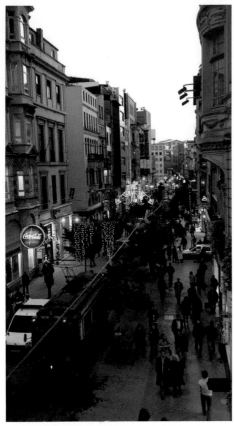

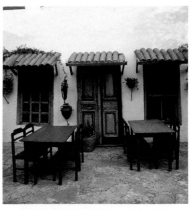

A welcoming café

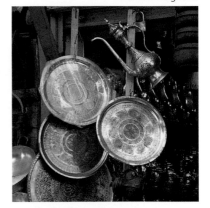

Pedestrian promenade in Beyoglu, Taksim

Shimmering copperwork

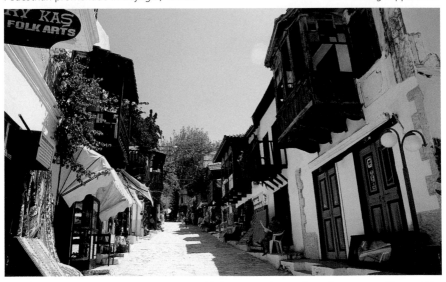

Weekly bazaar in the small Mediterranean village of Kas

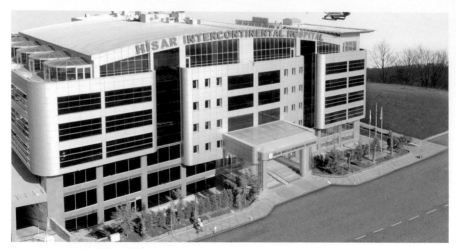

Hisar Intercontinental Hospital

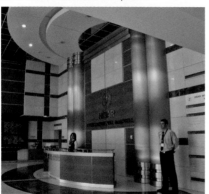

Main lobby

Hisar Intercontinental Hospital—"Providing preventive medicine, diagnostic, and treatment services combined with experience, modern technology, and international accreditation."

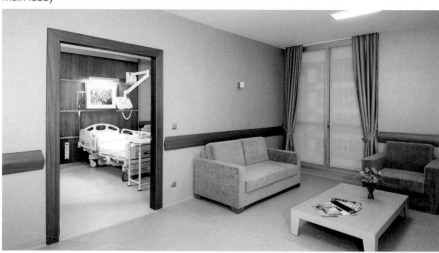

Spacious patient suite

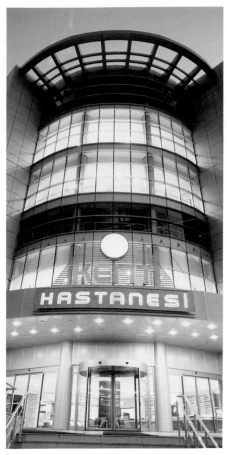

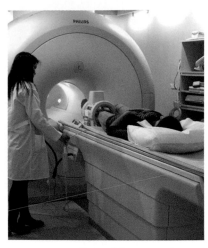

State-of-the-art equipment

Kent Hospital is the leading healthcare provider in the Aegean region.

Kent Hospital entrance

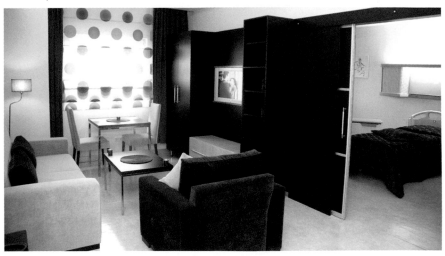

Luxurious patient suite

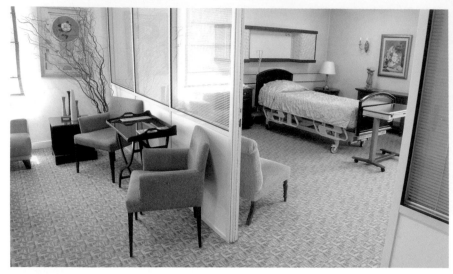

Istanbul Memorial Hospital patient room

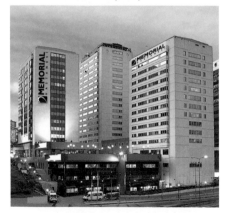

MHG main campus

Memorial Healthcare Group (MHG) offers high-quality healthcare services in every medical specialty for the international patient.

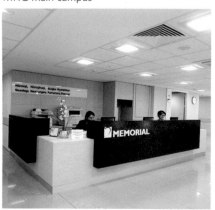

Polyclinics/outpatient area

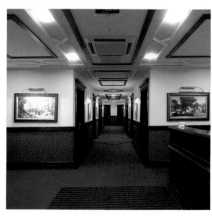

Memorial Hospital Guest House

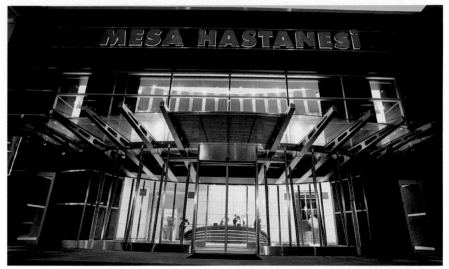

MESA Hospital

Adopting a patient-centered management philosophy, MESA Hospital strives to have its entire staff see things through their patients' (and their families') eyes.

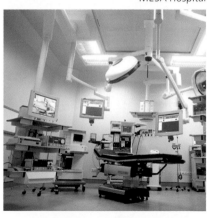

Modern equipment and facilities

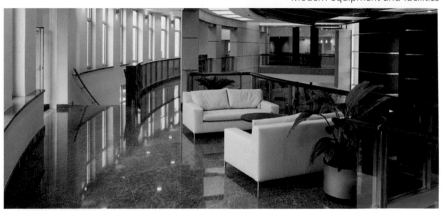

Contemporary and comfortable

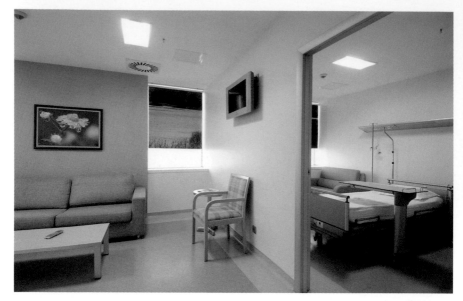

Inpatient room

Yeditepe University
Hospital offers an
International Services
Department to assist
patients with every
detail of their care.

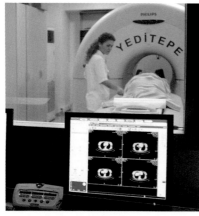

PET-CT nuclear medicine

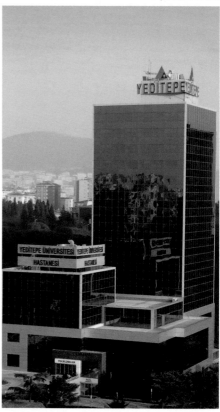

Yeditepe University Hospital

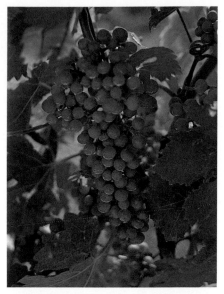
Wine tasting at Sirince vineyards

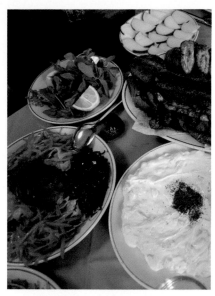
Delicious and healthful Turkish cuisine

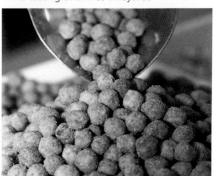
A major supplier of the world's nuts

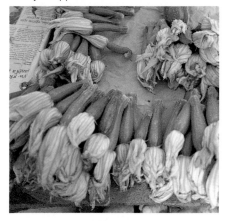
Acur, a special Turkish cucumber

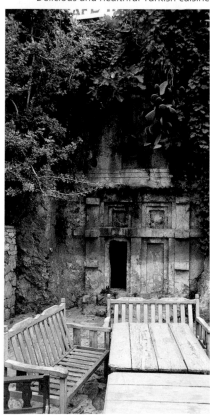
Historical relics in Dalyan

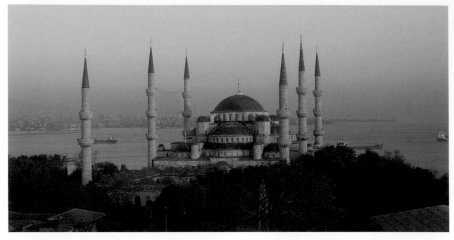
Sultanahmet Mosque

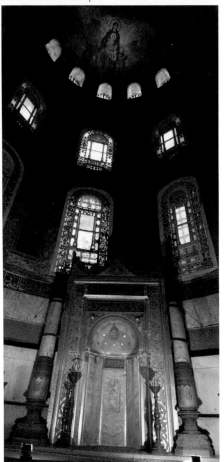

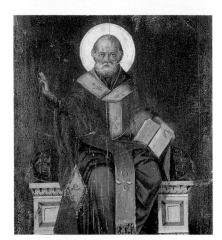
St. Nicholas Church, Demre, Antalya

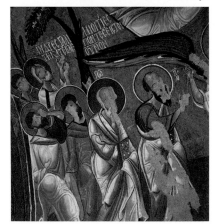

Interior view from Ayasofya Mosque

A close-up of magnificent mosaics

- *Borek* are pies of flaky pastry stuffed with meat, cheese, or potatoes. Grape leaves, cabbage leaves, and green peppers stuffed with spiced rice are all *dolma.*
- The best-known sweet pastries are *baklava* and *kadayif.* Other Turkish desserts are often milk based, such as *sutlac* (rice pudding), *tavuk gogsu* (a sweet that surprisingly contains the white meat of chicken), and *kazandibi* (caramelized pudding).
- Renowned Turkish coffee comes thick and dark in a small cup. *Raki,* which is made of anise and grapes, is a unique beverage that those who drink alcohol should try, but probably only once—only the strong can handle this "lion's milk."

Turkey's Cities of Health

Health travelers are attracted to Turkey for its world-class hospitals and medical services, most of which are centered in Istanbul, Ankara, and Izmir. Medical groups located in these cities offer both topnotch healthcare and pleasant touring experiences before and after treatment.

Istanbul

Istanbul welcomed more than 6.5 million tourists in 2007. Once named Byzantium and later Constantinople, Istanbul is Europe's most populous city, with 12 million inhabitants. The center of Turkey's cultural, economic, business, and social life, Istanbul is one of the most diverse and culturally rich cities in the world. It is located on the Bosphorus Strait and encompasses the natural harbor known as the Golden Horn. It is the only city in the world sited on two continents, and it has both European and Asian parts.

Istanbul's majestic mosques, churches, synagogues, and public buildings attest to its rich and varied history. The first human settlements in Istanbul date back to 5500–3500 BC. Later, Istanbul served as the capital city of the Roman Empire (330–395), the Byzantine Empire (395–1204 and 1261–1453), the Latin Empire (1204–1261), and the Ottoman Empire (1453–1922). The United Nations Educational, Scientific, and Cultural Organization (UNESCO) added the historic areas of Istanbul to its list of World Heritage Sites in 1985.

Among the hundreds of monuments scattered throughout the city, one of the finest standouts is Topkapi Palace, which was the official and primary residence of the Ottoman sultans for 400 years. Another is Hagia Sophia, once a patriarchal basilica—the largest cathedral in the world for nearly a thousand years—and later a mosque; now a museum, it is admired as an epitome of Byzantine architecture. Istanbul is also home to the famous Grand Bazaar, one of the largest covered markets in the world, encompassing more than 58 streets and 4,000 shops. Many of the stalls are grouped by type of goods, and feature jewelry, pottery, spices, carpets, leather, and more. The bazaar hosts 250,000–400,000 visitors daily.

Istanbul frequently hosts international festivals, conferences, and summits. The Fifth World Water Forum, for example, convened in Istanbul in March 2009; the annual meetings of the World Bank Group and the International Monetary Fund were held in Istanbul in October 2009. Thanks to its diverse cultural heritage and lively art scene, Istanbul was chosen as the joint European Capital of Culture for 2010.

Ankara

As the capital of Turkey, Ankara is the country's second largest city after Istanbul. It has a population of 4.4 million and an average elevation of 2,800 feet (850 meters). Centrally located in Anatolia, it is an important commercial and industrial city. The oldest settlements in and around Ankara's city center date to the Hattian civilization of the Bronze Age. Subsequently conquered in 25 BC by the emperor Augustus, the city then passed under the control of the Roman Empire.

Today Ankara is the center of the Turkish state and government, housing all foreign embassies. It is an important crossroads of trade, strategically located at the center of Turkey's highway and railway networks, and serves as the marketing center for the surrounding agricultural area. Ankara is also home to no less than ten universities.

Izmir

Historically called Smyrna, Izmir today is Turkey's third most populous city, with 3.7 million inhabitants. As the country's largest port after Istanbul, Izmir is the passageway for 20 percent of Turkish exports. Its Aegean shores are among the loveliest landscapes in the country—olive groves, rocky crags, and pinewoods surround the city. Reflecting its location in the westernmost part of the country, Izmir's citizens combine a Western lifestyle with

Turkish customs and habits. Izmir is widely regarded as one of Turkey's most progressive cities in its values, ideology, lifestyle, and dynamism.

Izmir represents almost 5,000 years of urban history. It incorporates several centers of international tourism, including Bodrum, Cesme, Foca, Kusadasi, and Mordogan, as well as the nearby ancient cities of Ephesus, Klazomenai, Pergamon, Sardis, and Troy. The modern city still retains traces of its ancient Ottoman and Levantine past; as the hub of the Levantine community, Izmir has long been a center of culture and civilization where Judaism, Christianity, and Islam have always coexisted peacefully.

Boasting numerous museums, concert halls, and sports events, along with five universities, Izmir is a sophisticated city of culture and arts and a top destination for vacationers. Every year the city hosts an international arts festival and the Izmir International Fair. Izmir hosted the World University Games (Universiade) in 2005.

The Medical Traveler's Essentials

This section provides a handy rundown of practical information on transportation, currency, communications, and other "nuts and bolts" of travel to Turkey.

Geography

Turkey is a transcontinental Eurasian nation. Asian Turkey, made up largely of Anatolia, is 97 percent of the country. The remainder, eastern Thrace or Rumelia in the Balkan Peninsula, is European Turkey. Asian and European Turkey are separated by the Istanbul Bosphorus, the Sea of Marmara, and the Dardanelles Bosphorus, which together form a water link between the Black Sea and the Mediterranean. Turkey is geographically divided into seven regions: Marmara, Aegean, Black Sea, Central Anatolia, Eastern Anatolia, Southeastern Anatolia, and Mediterranean.

Climate

The coastal areas of Turkey bordering the Mediterranean Sea have a temperate climate, with hot, dry summers and wet, mildly cold winters, but conditions can be much harsher in the more arid interior. Mountains close to the coast prevent Mediterranean influences from extending inland, giving the central Anatolian plateau a continental climate with sharply contrasting seasons. Winters on the plateau are especially severe. Temperatures from –22°F to –40°F (–30°C to –40°C) can occur in the mountainous areas in the east, and snow may lie on the ground 120 days of the year; in the west, winter temperatures average below 34°F (1°C). Summer temperatures are generally above 86°F (30°C) during the day.

Time Zone

Turkey is in the Eastern European Time Zone, two hours ahead of Greenwich Mean Time (GMT+2). Daylight Saving Time or Summer Time (GMT+3) begins on the last Sunday in March at 0100 and ends on the last Sunday in October at 0100.

Languages

The official language of Turkey is Turkish, but more than 30 minority languages and regional dialects are used. The most widely spoken foreign language is English, which is taught in the school curriculum. German, French, Italian, and Spanish translators are available in major cities.

Visas

Generally, travelers from Canada, the UK, and the US must have a visa to enter Turkey. Ordinary passport holders can obtain three-month multiple-entry visas upon arrival in the immigration/customs areas of Turkish airports and seaports. Travelers from most European countries are exempt from visa requirements for up to 90 days. However, there are exceptions, so it's best to check with your travel planner or the Turkish Embassy in your country to determine the rules and procedures that apply in your case.

Immunizations

The US Centers for Disease Control and Prevention (CDC) recommend that all international travelers stay up-to-date with routine immunizations, which include influenza, chickenpox (or varicella), polio, measles/mumps/rubella (MMR), and diphtheria/pertussis/tetanus (DPT). Although childhood diseases, such as measles, rarely occur in the US today, they are not uncommon in many parts of the world, so an unvaccinated traveler is at risk for infection.

The CDC also recommends that all travelers who might be exposed to blood or other body fluids through medical treatment be immunized against hepatitis B. Immunization against hepatitis A and boosters for typhoid and polio are recommended as well. Travelers to Turkey's major cities do not need to take medicines to prevent malaria; there is, however, some risk of malaria in the eastern, rural areas. For more information, check the CDC's Web site, wwwn.cdc.gov/travel/destinations/list.aspx.

Transportation

Air. Most international airlines offer regular flights from all major cities of the world to Turkey's international airports. The national carrier—Turkish Airlines—and various private airlines, such as Atlasjet, Onur Air, Pegasus, and SunExpress, offer regular flights to Adana, Ankara, Antalya, Dalaman, Istanbul, Izmir, and Trabzon.

Sea. In addition to the numerous Mediterranean cruises available, several foreign shipping companies offer regular passage services to Turkish port cities. Car and passenger ferry services are also available for certain coastal destinations.

Rail. Train journeys can be made directly between Istanbul and some of the major cities in Europe.

Bus. Regular coach services operate between Turkey and Austria, France, Germany, Greece, Iran, Iraq, Italy, Jordan, Kuwait, the Netherlands, Saudi Arabia, Switzerland, and Syria. Within Turkey, fairly comfortable buses serve the major cities on a regular schedule at reasonable prices, usually somewhere in the US$20–50 range. Some companies, such as Ulusoy and Varan, offer nonstop bus service with meals, beverage service, and wireless Internet access during travel.

Customs Regulations

All passengers may freely import the following items:

- 200 cigarettes and 50 cigars
- 1 liter of wine or spirits
- five bottles of perfume
- gifts up to the value of 255.65 euros (about US$360)
- electronic articles up to the value of 255.65 euros (about US$360)
- a reasonable quantity of coffee and tea

There is no limit on the import of foreign currencies, but imported currencies should be declared on arrival to avoid difficulties on departure. If you bring jewelry, media players, radios, tape recorders, or sporting guns (proof of gun ownership is required), these should be registered in your passport to ensure free export when you depart.

Items prohibited for export are antiques, cacao, coffee, grain products, spices, and tea. Travelers may freely export the following:

- 4.4 pounds (2 kilograms) or three cartons of local tobacco products
- 11 pounds (5 kilograms) of alcoholic beverages
- local drinks and foodstuffs up to a total value of TL100 (about US$65), each commodity not to exceed 11 pounds (5 kilograms)
- gift articles up to a value of TL5,000 (about US$3,250)

Currency

The Republic of Turkey's unit of currency is the Turkish lira (TL); a lira is divided into 100 kurus. Paper money comes in TL denominations of 200, 100, 50, 20, 10, and 5. Coin denominations are TL1 and 50, 25, 10, and 5 kurus.

Telecommunications

Turkey's telecommunications network is undergoing rapid modernization and expansion, especially in mobile-cellular services. The official telecommunications center is Turk Telekom. Other private operators include Avea, Turkcell, and Vodafone. Inexpensive calling cards are available in shops and convenience stores.

International phone calls. The country code for Turkey is 90. When calling Turkey from another country, dial the appropriate international access code, followed by 90, then the area code, and then the number itself. When calling another country from Turkey, dial 00, followed by the appropriate country code, and then the area code and number.

Phone calls within Turkey. When calling major cities in Turkey, dial 0, followed by the area code and the number you're calling.

Area Codes

- Adana: 322
- Ankara: 312
- Antalya: 242
- Bursa: 224
- Istanbul Asya (Asia): 216
- Istanbul Avrupa (Europe): 212
- Izmir: 232

Useful Telephone Numbers

- Fire emergency: 110
- Health emergency: 112
- Registration for international calls: 115
- How to make calls: 118
- Addresses/zip codes: 119
- Phone problems: 121
- Police emergency: 155
- Directory assistance: 11811

Tipping

The American practice of overtipping is driving expectations up, but tipping guidelines in Turkey are still generally modest. It's best to tip in lira, although paper money (not coins) in other currencies is acceptable. In restaurants, small tips of 5–10 percent are appreciated, but not mandatory; in luxury restaurants, tip 10–15 percent. Porters in hotels and airports expect tips of about TL2–3 per bag. Don't tip taxi drivers; just round the fare upward to the next whole lira. (All taxis are metered, and payment should be based on the meter charge.)

General Business Hours

Government	Open weekdays	0830–1230, 1330–1730
Businesses	Open weekdays	0830/0900–1730
Department stores	Open daily	0900–2100
Shops	Open every day except New Year's Day	0900/1000–2100/2200
Convenience stores	Open daily	24 hours a day
Restaurants	Most open daily	0900–2300/2400

Electricity

Turkey operates on 220 volts, 50 Hz, with round-prong European-style plugs. Four- and five-star hotels often provide North American–style 120-volt, 60-Hz flush-mounted sockets (points) for North American flat-prong plugs. It's wise to travel with a small transformer and a set of plug adapters. And do read the fine print on any plug-in devices you take along. If you find yourself stuck without the right equipment, you'll find modern electrical appliance shops in all large Turkish cities and many smaller ones, too.

Smoking

Health travelers are advised not to smoke. In Turkey, as of July 2009, smoking is banned in cafés, restaurants, bars, and all public transportation, including taxis, trains, and boats.

Dress Code

Turkey is a predominantly Muslim country, and modest dress is the norm. Save short shorts, tank tops, bikinis, and miniskirts for the beach. Outside of cities, women should take notice of their surroundings and dress accordingly. In general, the more rural the area, the more conservative the standards of dress. At religious sites, women may be expected to cover their heads with a scarf.

Embassies and Consulates

It's a good idea to take information with you on the location and telephone number of your nation's embassy or consulate. You may need to contact its offices should you lose a passport or encounter some other difficulty while in Turkey. Here are a few of the offices typically contacted by travelers from English-speaking countries:

- Australian Consulate in Istanbul: 90 212 243.1333
- Australian Embassy in Ankara: 90 312 459.9550
- British Consulate in Istanbul: 90 212 334.6400
- British Embassy in Ankara: 90 312 409.2700
- Canadian Consulate in Istanbul: 90 212 251.9838
- Canadian Embassy in Ankara: 90 312 409.2700
- US Consulate General in Istanbul: 90 212 335.9000
- US Embassy in Ankara: 90 312 455.5555

Accommodations:
Recovery Lodgings and Hotels

The major commercial centers and tourist destinations of Turkey abound with family-owned and -operated *pensiones*, small
hotels, and modest guesthouses that are clean, quiet, and inexpensive. If you prefer local color to large, luxury accommodations—and if your recuperative needs are moderate—you may
wish to consider arranging such housing. We list here only a few
of the recovery lodges and hotels recommended by the hospitals
featured in Part Two of this book.

HOSPITAL GUESTHOUSES

Anadolu Medical Center Guest House	Anadolu Cad. No. 1
	Bayramoglu, Cikisi
	Cayirova Mevkii, Gebze
	Istanbul, TURKEY 41400
	Tel: 90 262 444.4276
	Fax: 90 262 654.0055
	Email: guest@anadolumedicalcenter.org

Memorial Hospital Guest House	Piyale Pasa Bulv. Memorial Center, A Blok Kat. 13 Okmeydani, Sisli Istanbul, TURKEY 34385 Tel: 90 212 320.6600 Fax: 90 212 320.0053 Email: info@memorialkonukevi.com; konukevi@memorial.com.tr Web: www.memorial.com.tr/eng/konukevi.php

RECOVERY LODGES AND SPAS

Balcova Thermal Hotel	Balcova Termal Balcova Izmir, TURKEY 35330 Tel: 90 232 259.0102 Fax: 90 232 259.0829 Email: info@balcovatermal.com Web: www.balcovatermal.com
Evital Private Rehabilitation Center	Eczacibasi Health Services Kosuyolu Cad. Cenap Sahabettin Sok. No. 84 Kosuyolu Istanbul, TURKEY 34718 Tel: 90 216 547.2500 Fax: 90 216 545.2503 Email: evital@evital.com.tr Web: www.evital.com.tr/en
Gural Sapanca Wellness Park	Tepebasi Mah. Sehit Cevdet Koc Cad. No. 73 Kirkpinar, Sapanca Sakarya, TURKEY 54600 Tel: 90 264 592.3030 Fax: 90 264 592.0932 Email: info@guralsapanca.com Web: www.guralsapanca.com

| Richmond Nua Wellness Spa | Rustem Pasa Mah. Sahil Yolu Cad. Sapanca, Sakarya Adapazari, TURKEY 54600 Tel: 90 264 582.2100 Fax: 90 264 582.2101 Email: richmondnua@richmondnua.com Web: www.richmondnua.com |

HOTELS: ISTANBUL

Bostanci Hotel	Mehmet Sevki Pasa Cad. No. 20 Bostanci Istanbul, TURKEY 34744 Tel: 90 216 362.4848 Fax: 90 216 372.6000 Email: info@thebostancihotel.com Web: www.thebostancihotel.com
Ciragan Palace Kempinski Istanbul	Ciragan Cad. 32 Besiktas Istanbul, TURKEY 34349 Tel: 90 212 326.4646 Fax: 90 212 259.6687 Email: reservationoffice.ciraganpalace @kempinski.com Web: www.kempinski-istanbul.com
Dedeman Hotel	Yildiz Posta Cad. 50 Esentepe Istanbul, TURKEY 34340 Tel: 90 212 337.4500 Fax: 90 212 275.1100 Email: istanbul@dedeman.com Web: www.dedeman.com
Four Seasons Hotel Istanbul at the Bosphorus	Ciragan Cad. No. 28 Besiktas Istanbul, TURKEY 34349 Tel: 90 212 381.4000 Fax: 90 212 381.4010 Web: www.fourseasons.com/bosphorus

Four Seasons Hotel Istanbul at Sultanahmet	Tevkifhane Sok. No. 1 Sultanahmet, Eminonu Istanbul, TURKEY 34110 Tel: 90 212 402.3000 Fax: 90 212 402.3010 Web: www.fourseasons.com/istanbul
Grand Cevahir Hotel	Darulaceze Cad. No. 9 Okmeydani, Sisli Istanbul, TURKEY 34382 Tel: 90 212 314.4242 Fax: 90 212 314.4244 Email: info@grandcevahirhotel.com.tr Web: www.grandcevahirhotel.com
Green Park Merter	Nazim Erten Sok. No. 13 Merter Istanbul, TURKEY 34173 Tel: 90 212 507.7373 Fax: 90 212 642.4444 Email: merterrezervasyon@thegreenpark.com Web: www.thegreenpark.com
Hilton Istanbul	Cumhuriyet Cad. Harbiye Istanbul, TURKEY 34367 Tel: 90 212 315.6000 Fax: 90 212 240.4165 Email: sales.istanbul@hilton.com Web: www1.hilton.com
History Hotel Istanbul	Gencturk Cad. Sirvanizade Sok. No. 14 Sehzadebasi Istanbul, TURKEY 34470 Tel: 90 212 520.6607 Fax: 90 212 520.6611 Email: info@historyhotel.com Web: www.historyhotel.com

Hotel Bostanci Prenses	Bostanci Degirmen Yolu Cad. No. 24 Istanbul, TURKEY 34752 Tel: 90 216 577.2600 Fax: 90 216 577.2616 Email: info@hotelbostanciprenses.com Web: www.hotelbostanciprenses.com
Hotel Byotell Istanbul	Saniye Ermutlu Sok. No. 3 Kozyatagi, Kadikoy Istanbul, TURKEY 34742 Tel: 90 216 571.6100 Fax: 90 216 571.6110 Email: sales@byotell.com.tr Web: www.byotell.com.tr
Hotel Ibis Istanbul	Kazlicesme Mah. Kennedy Cad. No. 56 Zeytinburnu Istanbul, TURKEY 34025 Tel: 90 212 414.3900 Fax: 90 212 414.3929 Email: h5998@accor.com Web: www.ibishotel.com
Hotel Nova	Rihtim Cad. Kirmizi Kusak Sok. No. 12 Kadikoy Istanbul, TURKEY 34710 Tel: 90 216 550.0351 Fax: 90 216 550.0392 Email: nova@istanbulnovahotel.com Web: www.istanbulnovahotel.com
Hyatt Regency Istanbul	Taskisla Cad. No. 1 Taksim Istanbul, TURKEY 34437 Tel: 90 212 368.1234 Fax: 90 212 368.1000 Email: istanbul.regency@hyatt.com Web: http://istanbul.regency.hyatt.com

Istanbul Marriott Hotel Asia	Kayisdagi Cad. No. 1/1 Atasehir Istanbul, TURKEY 34750 Tel: 90 216 570.0000 Fax: 90 216 469.9999 Email: melike.karakan@marriotthotels.com Web: www.marriott.com
Marmara Camlica	Atif Bey Sok. No. 67–69 Acibadem Istanbul, TURKEY 34662 Tel: 90 216 362.1010 Fax: 90 212 292.3321 Email: residence-info@themarmarahotels.com Web: www.themarmarahotels.com
Marmara Pendik	Sahil Yolu Ankara Cad. No. 239 Alt Kaynarca, Pendik Istanbul, TURKEY 34890 Tel: 90 216 362.1010 Fax: 90 216 362.8375 Email: residence-info@themarmarahotels.com Web: www.themarmarahotels.com
Ramada Plaza Istanbul	Halaskargazi Cad. No. 63 Osmanbey, Sisli Istanbul, TURKEY 34373 Tel: 90 212 315.4444 Fax: 90 212 315.4445 Email: info@ramadaplazaistanbul.com Web: www.ramadaplazaistanbul.com
Renaissance Polat Istanbul Hotel	Sahil Yolu Cad. No. 2 Yesilyurt Istanbul, TURKEY 34149 Tel: 90 212 414.1800 Fax: 90 212 414.1970 Email: rezervasyon@polatholding.com Web: www.marriott.com

Ritz-Carlton Istanbul	Suzer Plaza, Elmadag Askerocagi Cad. No. 15 Sisli Istanbul, TURKEY 34367 Tel: 90 212 334.4444 Fax: 90 212 334.4455 Web: www.ritzcarlton.com
Sofa Hotel and Residence	Tesvikiye Cad. No. 41–41A Nisantasi, Sisli Istanbul, TURKEY 34367 Tel: 90 212 368.1818 Fax: 90 212 291.9117 Email: info@thesofahotel.com Web: www.thesofahotel.com
Suadiye Princess Hotel	Plaj Yolu Sok. No. 51 Suadiye, Kadikoy Istanbul, TURKEY 34740 Tel: 90 212 386.3119; 90 212 225.4204 Fax: 90 212 291.7239 Email: info@hotelsuadiye.com Web: www.hotelsuadiye.com
Surmeli Hotel	Prof. Dr. Bulent Tarcan Sok. No. 3 Gayrettepe Istanbul, TURKEY 34349 Tel: 90 212 272.1161 Fax: 90 212 272.0516 Email: salesistanbul@surmelihotels.com Web: www.surmelihotels.com
Swissotel The Bosphorus, Istanbul	Bayildim Cad. No. 2 Macka, Besiktas Istanbul, TURKEY 34357 Tel: 90 212 326.1100 Fax: 90 212 326.1122 Email: istanbul@swissotel.com Web: www.istanbul.swissotel.com

Tuzla Apart Hotel	Sahil Yolu Sehitler Cad. No. 31 Tuzla Istanbul, TURKEY 34740 Tel: 90 216 395.8840 Fax: 90 216 395.8854 Email: info@tuzlaaparthotel.com Web: www.tuzlaaparthotel.com

HOTELS: KOCAELI

Bayramoglu Resort Hotel	Piri Reis Mah. Bayramoglu Cad. No. 229 Bayramoglu Kocaeli, TURKEY 41870 Tel: 90 262 653.4030 Fax: 90 262 653.4033 Email: info@bayramogluresort.com Web: www.bayramogluresort.com
Hotel Hegsagone	Balyanoz Koyu Kaptan Sok. No. 13/1 Bayramoglu, Gebze Kocaeli, TURKEY 41870 Tel: 90 262 653.5959 Fax: 90 262 653.8549 Email: hotel@hegsagone.com Web: www.hegsagone.com
Yelkenkaya Hotel	Piri Reis Mah. Yelkenkaya Cad. No. 69 Bayramoglu, Gebze Kocaeli, TURKEY 41700 Tel: 90 262 653.8800 Fax: 90 262 653.2889 Email: info@otelyelkenkaya.com Web: www.otelyelkenkaya.com

HOTELS: ANKARA

Ankara Best Hotel	Ataturk Bulv. No. 195 Kavaklidere Ankara, TURKEY 06680 Tel: 90 312 467.0880 Fax: 90 312 467.0885 Email: reservation@besthotel.com.tr Web: www.besthotel.com.tr
Ankara Hilton SA Hotel	Tahran Cad. No. 12 Kavaklidere Ankara, TURKEY 06700 Tel: 90 312 455.0000 Fax: 90 312 455.0055 Email: sales.ankara@hilton.com Web: www1.hilton.com
Bilkent Hotel	Universiteler Mah. 1599 Sok. No. 6 Bilkent Ankara, TURKEY 06800 Tel: 90 312 266.4686 Fax: 90 312 266.4679 Email: info@bilkentotel.com.tr Web: www.bilkentotel.com.tr
Gazi Park Hotel	Bestepeler Mah. 1 Cad. No. 51 Sogutozu Ankara, TURKEY 06530 Tel: 90 312 215.6666 Fax: 90 312 212.2108 Email: contact@gaziparkhotel.com Web: www.gaziparkhotel.com
Rescate Boutique Hotel	Rabindranath Tagore Cad. (4 Cad.) No. 80 Yildiz Ankara, TURKEY 06560 Tel: 90 312 442.6506 Fax: 90 312 442.9565 Email: info@rescatehotel.com Web: www.rescatehotel.com

HOTELS: IZMIR

Hilton Izmir	Gazi Osmanpasa Bulv. No. 7 Izmir, TURKEY 35210 Tel: 90 232 497.6060 Fax: 90 232 497.6000 Email: sales.izmir@hilton.com Web: www1.hilton.com
Izmir Palas Hotel	Ataturk Bulv. Izmir, TURKEY 35210 Tel: 90 232 465.0030 Fax: 90 232 422.6870 Email: info@izmirpalas.com.tr Web: www.izmirpalas.com.tr
Izmir Princess Hotel	Ilica Mah. Zeytin Sok. No. 112 Narlidere Izmir, TURKEY 35331 Tel: 90 232 238.5151 Fax: 90 232 239.0939 Email: izmirprincess@izmirprincess.com.tr Web: www.izmirprincess.com.tr
Mövenpick Hotel Izmir	Cumhuriyet Bulv. 138 Izmir, TURKEY 35210 Tel: 90 232 488.1414 Fax: 90 232 484.8070 Email: hotel.izmir@moevenpick.com Web: www.moevenpick-hotels.com
Ontur Izmir Boutique Hotel	Lamet Kaplan Mah. Gazi Bulv. No. 130 Izmir, TURKEY 35241 Tel: 90 232 425.8181 Fax: 90 232 425.8787 Email: izmirinfo@onturhotels.com Web: www.onturhotels.com

Sisus Hotel	Dalyankoy Yat Limani Cesme Izmir, TURKEY 35550 Tel: 90 232 724.0330 Fax: 90 232 724.9656 Email: info@sisushotel.com Web: www.sisushotel.com
Swissotel Grand Efes, Izmir	Gaziosmanpasa Bulv. No. 1 Alsancak Izmir, TURKEY 35210 Tel: 90 232 414.0000 Fax: 90 232 414.1010 Email: izmir@swissotel.com Web: www.swissotel.com/izmir

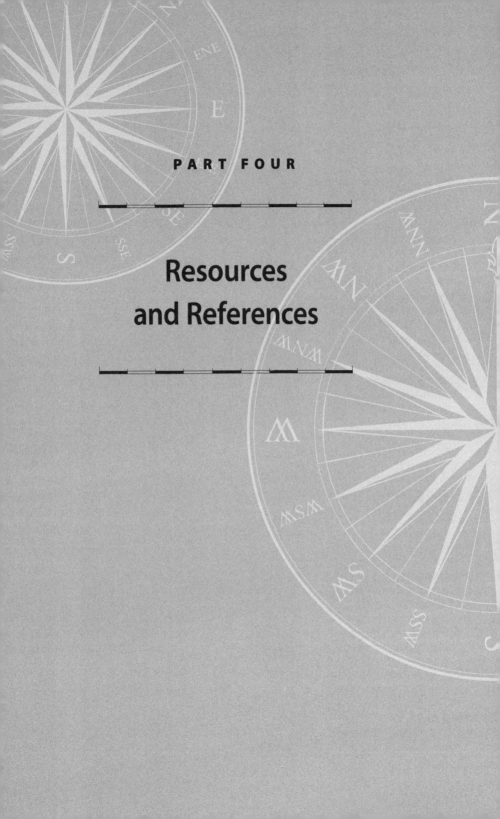

PART FOUR

Resources
and References

ADDITIONAL RESOURCES

Other Editions of *Patients Beyond Borders*

The international *Patients Beyond Borders: Second Edition* explores medical travel's practical and personal considerations and provides information on the specialties, hospitals, and accommodations currently offered to medical travelers in 21 countries. Each year Healthy Travel Media also publishes new, specialized editions of *Patients Beyond Borders*. Country-specific editions include India, Korea, Malaysia, Singapore, Taiwan, and Thailand. Visit www.patientsbeyond borders.com to check on special editions for your destination.

World, Country, and City Information

The World Factbook. Compiled by the US Central Intelligence Agency (CIA) and cataloged by country, this is an excellent source of general, up-to-date information about the geography, economy, and history of countries around the world. Go to www.cia.gov, find "Library and Reference" in the left column, and click on "The World Factbook."

Lonely Planet. Lonely Planet's books are arguably the most comprehensive and reliable guides for both budget and luxury travelers. The series covers every country and city destination featured in *Patients Beyond Borders*. Increasingly, its published information is being posted online as well, at www.lonelyplanet.com.

Becoming Informed Here and Abroad

You: The Smart Patient: An Insider's Guide for Getting the Best Treatment.** Physicians Michael F. Roizen and Mehmet C. Oz have written a witty, often irreverent, and highly useful guide to becoming an informed patient, whether in your doctor's office or dentist's chair, on the surgeon's table, or in an emergency room. This 400-page consumer bible is packed with information on patients' rights, surgical precautions, second and third opinions, health insurance plans, health records, and precautionary advice that falls outside the scope of this book.

World Travel Guide. The publishers of the *Columbus World Travel Guide* also sponsor www.worldtravelguide.net, which offers good information on countries and major metropolitan areas throughout the world. Go to the Web site's "Choose Guide" search to find information on airports, tours, attractions, cruises, and more.

Google Earth. If you've not downloaded Google Earth, go to http://earth.google .com/ and do so. It's truly one of the wonders of the online world. After you follow the download instructions, you can zoom to your home's rooftop or "fly" to any continent, country, or city on the planet simply by typing in the appropriate keywords. Legends include city names, roads, terrain, populated places, borders, 3-D buildings, and more.

Information about Turkey

- "Turkey's Medical Tourism Potential," by Adam Bahattin, *Medical Tourism Magazine,* January/February 2009, pp. 42–45.
- *OECD (Organization for Economic Cooperation and Development) Health Data 2008: How Does Turkey Compare,* www.oecd.org/ dataoecd/46/5/38980477.pdf
- Ministry of Health official Web site, www.saglik.gov.tr
- Ministry of Foreign Affairs official Web site, www.mfa.gov.tr
- Visa Information for Foreigners, www.mfa.gov.tr/visa-information -for-foreigners.en.mfa
- Ministry of Culture and Tourism official Web site, www.turizm.gov.tr
- Traveling to Turkey, www.goturkey .com

- YASED: International Investors Association of Turkey official Web site, www.yased.org.tr

Passports and Visas

Travisa. Dozens of online agencies offer visa services—but we've found this agency, at www.travisa.com, to be reliable and accessible by telephone as well. Travisa offers good customer service and followup. Their Web site also carries links to information on immunization requirements, travel warnings, current weather, and more.

Currency Converter

www.xe.com. To learn quickly how much your money is worth in your country of interest, go to this site and click on "Quick Currency Converter."

Traveler's Tips

Smart Packing by Susan Foster (Third Edition, Smart Travel Press, 2008) includes timely information on airport security, airline regulations, and travel security. It offers advice on luggage selection, matching clothes to the occasion, and finding the right fabrics and styles for every season. The book also includes chapters on how to travel light and what to do about toiletries, cosmetics, electrical appliances, and travel gadgets.

International Hospital Accreditation

Joint Commission International (JCI). Mentioned frequently throughout this book, JCI remains the only game in town for international hospital accreditation. To see a current list of accredited hospitals by country, go to www.joint commissioninternational.org.

Medical Information

MedlinePlus is a US government–sponsored site that brings together a wealth of information from such sources as the National Library of Medicine (the world's largest medical library), the National Institutes of Health, *Merriam-Webster's Medical Dictionary* (see below), and the *United States Pharmacopeia*. Go to http://medlineplus.gov and click on any of the choices in the left column. The online tour at www.nlm.nih.gov/medline plus/tour/medlineplustour.html helps you navigate this massive site.

Merriam-Webster's Medical Dictionary.

If a multisyllabic medical term stumps you, don't run out and purchase an un-abridged brick of a medical dictionary—several free, online medical glossaries offer more than you probably want to know on most health topics. *Merriam-Webster's Medical Dictionary* is provided on a number of sites, including Medline-Plus (see above) and InteliHealth (www.intelihealth.com). The simplest access is through http://dictionary.reference.com. Just type in a medical word or phrase, and voila! For a richer exploration, Medi-cineNet (www.medicinenet.com) and similar sources offer articles, services, and a thicket of sponsored links.

Medical Travel Resources

World Health Organization (WHO). On its official Web site at www.who.int, WHO provides profiles of member countries, overviews of significant health topics, and statistics of interest to health travelers and medical professional worldwide.

Medical Nomad. A group of medical professionals, technology geeks, and consultants established www.medical nomad.com in 2004 to bring together an impressive body of information, including specific data on treatments, clinics, physicians, accreditation, and other topics of interest to the health traveler. Medical Nomad's extensive database allows readers to search by procedure, provider, and destination, with clinic and country summaries as well as lay summaries of common treatments.

RevaHealth is a searchable database of healthcare providers around the world. At www.revahealth.com, the unique directory system and powerful search engine allow patients to find detailed information easily. For example, RevaHealth has a long list of dentists in Turkey at www.revahealth.com/dentists/turkey. The platform also lets patients select providers and talk to them directly for a consultation.

International Society of Travel Medicine (ISTM).

If you're looking for information about immunizations, infectious diseases, or other aspects of medical travel, check out the ISTM Web site at www.istm.org. This organization maintains offices in Georgia, US, and in Munich, Germany, to promote safe and healthy travel and to facilitate education, service, and research activities in the field of travel medicine. Most useful to the health traveler is the society's searchable database of travel medicine practitioners and clinics.

Medical Tourism Insight is a monthly online newsletter written for the medical travel industry as well as employers, benefits managers, government officials, and prospective patients. Coverage includes objective and timely information on overseas medical care and related issues, such as health insurance and employee health benefits. The Web site is www.medical tourisminsight.com.

International Medical Travel Journal (IMTJ). *IMTJ* is the world's leading journal for the medical travel industry. While geared more toward industry professionals than consumers, it does provide a free online guide for potential patients at www.imtjonline.com. There's a free email newsletter, too, and a paid subscription service for those who are serious about industry news.

Beauty from Afar. If you're seeking more specialized information on cosmetic/aesthetic surgery or dental care, author and medical traveler Jeff Schult can fill you in on the main destinations, leading clinics and facilities, and third-party agents. Published in 2006 (Stewart, Tabori & Chang), this 224-page paperback is written in an anecdotal style, providing numerous firsthand accounts that give prospective patients a thorough perspective on the health travel experience.

Medical Tourism in Developing Countries, by Milica Z. Bookman and Karla R. Bookman (Palgrave Macmillan, 2007), explores the international marketplace for medical services and its potential for developing countries. While it's more an academic work than a consumer guide, physicians, administrators, and healthcare officials will find this book's economic perspective and vast bank of data on the industry instructive.

Refining Your Internet Research

The Google Guide. While you may not wish to become a wild-eyed expert on the nuances of search engines, a little additional knowledge can greatly enhance your efficiency in narrowing your health travel choices. Consultant and Internet search guru Nancy Blachman (coauthor of *How to Do Everything with Google*) has posted a useful online tutorial entitled "The Google Guide." Go to www.googleguide.com, click on "Novice," and you'll find a wealth of information on conducting Internet searches that will greatly improve your online health travel quests. Most of this information applies to other search engines as well, including Yahoo, MSN, and AOL.

MEDICAL GLOSSARY

Many medical terms are used in this book. The following is a list of the most commonly used terms. For further information, please consult your doctor.

Acute-care. Providing emergency services and general medical and surgical treatment for sudden severe disorders (as compared with long-term care for chronic illness).

Addiction. Occurs when a person has no control over the use of a substance, such as drugs or alcohol. Also includes addictions to food, gambling, and sex.

Aesthetics. A general term for medical treatments and surgical procedures undertaken to improve appearance. Such procedures include (but are not limited to) facelifts, tummy tucks, laser resurfacing of skin, Botox injection, cosmetic dentistry, and others.

Alzheimer's disease. A degenerative disorder of neurons in the brain that disrupts thought, perception, and behavior.

Anesthesia. Loss of physical sensation produced by sedation. Anesthesia may be given as (1) general, which affects the entire body and is accompanied by loss of consciousness; (2) regional, which affects an entire area of the body; and (3) local, which affects a limited part of the body (usually superficial).

Angiography. An x-ray procedure that uses dye injected into the coronary arteries to study circulation in the heart.

Angioplasty. A procedure that uses a tiny balloon on the end of a catheter to widen blocked or constricted arteries in the heart.

Arthroscopy or arthroscopic surgery. The use of a tubelike instrument utilizing fiber optics to examine, treat, or perform surgery on a joint.

Bariatric. Pertaining to the control and treatment of obesity and allied diseases.

Birmingham hip resurfacing (BHR). A surgically implanted metal-on-metal hip joint replacement system. It is called a resurfacing prosthesis because only the surface of the femoral head (ball) is removed to implant the femoral component.

Bone densitometry. A method of measuring bone strength, used to diagnose osteoporosis.

Botox. A nonsurgical, physician-administered injection treatment to temporarily reduce moderate to severe wrinkles on the face.

Cardiac. Pertaining to the heart.

Cardiac catheterization. The insertion of a catheter into the arteries of the heart to diagnose heart disease. See also **angiography.**

Cardiothoracic. Pertaining to the heart and the chest.

Cardiovascular. Pertaining to the heart and blood vessels that make up the circulatory system. See also **vascular surgery.**

Cataract. Cloudiness of the lens in the eye, which affects vision. Cataracts, which often occur in older people, can be corrected with surgery to replace the damaged lens with an artificial plastic lens known as an intraocular lens.

Colonoscopy. An examination of the interior of the colon, using a thin, lighted tube (a colonoscope) inserted into the rectum.

Computed tomography (CT). Sometimes known as CAT scanning. A noninvasive diagnostic tool that uses x-rays to provide cross-sectional images of the body. Used to detect cancer, determine heart function, and provide images of body organs. May be used in conjunction with **positron emission tomography (PET).**

Coronary artery bypass graft (CABG). Surgical procedure to create alternative paths for blood to flow around obstructions in the coronary arteries, most often using arteries or veins from other parts of the body.

Cosmetic surgery. Plastic surgery undertaken to improve appearance. See also **aesthetics** and **plastic surgery.**

Craniofacial. Pertaining to the head and face.

CyberKnife. A tool for radiosurgery that delivers precise high-dose radiation. Can be used for tumors of the pancreas, liver, lungs, and brain.

Diabetes. A chronic disease characterized by abnormally high levels of sugar in the blood.

Discectomy. Removal of all or part of an intervertebral disc (a soft structure that acts as a shock absorber between two bones in the spine).

Electrocardiogram (EKG or ECG). A diagnostic test that measures the heart's electrical activity.

Endocrinology. The branch of medicine that studies hormonal systems and treats disorders that arise when hormones are out of balance.

Endoscope. A slender, tubular optical instrument used as a viewing system for examining an inner part of the body and, with an attached instrument, for performing surgery or detecting tumors.

Extracorporeal shock wave therapy (ESWT). A noninvasive treatment that involves delivery of shock waves to a painful area.

Gamma Knife. A form of radiation therapy that focuses low-dose gamma radiation on a precise target, such as a tumor of the brain or breast.

Gastroenterology. The branch of medicine that studies and treats disorders of the digestive system.

Genetics. The study of inheritance.

Gynecology. The branch of medicine that studies and treats females, especially pertaining to their reproductive system.

Hematology. The study of the nature, function, and diseases of the blood and of blood-forming organs.

Hemopoietic or hematopoietic. Pertaining to the formation of blood.

Hepatitis. Inflammation of the liver caused by a virus or toxin. There are different forms of viral hepatitis. Vaccines are available for hepatitis A and B. There is no vaccine for hepatitis C.

Hepatobiliary. Pertaining to the bile ducts.

Hepatology. The branch of medicine that studies and treats disorders of the liver.

Holter monitor. A wearable electronic device used to obtain a continuous recording of the heart's electrical activity. See **electrocardiogram (EKG or ECG).**

Immunization. Inoculation with a vaccine to render a person resistant to a disease.

Immunology. The branch of medicine that studies and treats disorders of the body's mechanisms for fighting disease, especially infectious diseases.

Implant. *In dentistry:* a small metal pin placed inside the jawbone to mimic the root of a tooth. Dental implants can be used to help anchor a false tooth, a crown, or a bridge. *In fertility treatment:* to place an embryo in the uterus.

Intensive Care Unit (ICU). The hospital ward in which 24-hour specialized nursing and monitoring are provided for patients who are critically ill or have undergone major surgical procedures.

International Organization for Standardization (ISO). An organization based in Geneva, Switzerland, that approves and accredits the facilities and administrations of hospitals and clinics but not their practices, procedures, or methods.

Intracytoplasmic sperm injection (ICSI). A type of fertility treatment in which a single sperm cell is inserted into an egg using special micromanipulation equipment.

Intrauterine insemination (IUI). Introduction of prepared sperm (either the male partner's or a donor's) into the uterus to improve chances of pregnancy.

In vitro fertilization (IVF). Known as the test-tube baby technique. Eggs are fertilized outside the body, and then embryos are introduced back into the woman's uterus.

Joint Commission International (JCI). The international affiliate accreditation agency of the Joint Commission. JCI inspects and accredits healthcare providers worldwide using US-based standards.

Laparoscope. A thin, lighted tube used to examine and treat tissues and organs inside the abdomen.

LAP-BAND. An adjustable silicone band inserted laparoscopically around the upper part of the stomach, thereby reducing the stomach's food storage area and promoting weight loss.

LASIK (laser-assisted *in situ* keratomileusis). A laser procedure to reduce dependency on eyeglasses or contact lenses by permanently changing the shape of the cornea, the clear covering of the front of the eye.

Liposuction. The surgical withdrawal of fat from under the skin, using a small incision and suctioning.

Lithotripsy. A procedure that breaks up kidney stones or gallstones using sound waves. Also called extracorporeal shock wave lithotripsy (ESWL).

Magnetic resonance imaging (MRI). A noninvasive diagnostic tool that uses a large magnet, radio waves, and a computer to produce clear images of the interior of the body. Used to diagnose spine and joint problems, heart disease, and cancer.

Mammography. X-ray imaging of the breast for detection of cancer.

Maxillofacial. Pertaining to the jaws and face.

Microsurgical epididymal sperm aspiration (MESA). Obtaining immature sperm cells from the epididymis (which joins the testicle to the vas deferens), in cases where obstruction in the genital tract leads to absence of sperm in the ejaculate. The recovered sperm can be used for **intracytoplasmic sperm injection (ICSI).**

Minimal access surgery. Also called minimally invasive surgery. Any of a variety of approaches used to reduce the trauma of surgery and to speed recovery. These approaches include "keyhole" surgery, endoscopy, arthroscopy, laparoscopy, or the use of small incisions.

Myocardial infarction (MI). Heart attack.

Neonatology. The branch of medicine specializing in the care and treatment of newborns.

Nephrology. The branch of medicine that studies and treats disorders of the kidneys.

Neurology. The branch of medicine that studies and treats disorders of the nervous system, including the brain.

Neuro-oncology. The branch of medicine that studies and treats cancers of the nervous system.

Neuro-ophthalmology. The branch of medicine that studies and treats disorders of the nerves in the eye.

Neurosurgery. Surgery on the brain or other parts of the nervous system.

Obstetrics. The branch of medicine focusing on pregnancy and childbirth.

Oncology. The branch of medicine that studies and treats cancer.

Ophthalmology. The branch of medicine that studies and treats disorders of the eye.

Orthodontics. The branch of dentistry focusing on the prevention and correction of irregular tooth positioning, as by means of braces.

Orthopedics. The branch of medicine that studies and treats diseases and injuries of the bones and joints.

Osteoporosis. Thinning of the bones and reduction in bone mass, which increases the risk of fractures and decreases mobility, especially in the elderly.

Otorhinolaryngology. The branch of medicine that studies and treats ear, nose, and throat disorders.

Pacemaker. An electronic device surgically implanted into a patient's chest to regulate the heartbeat.

Parkinson's disease. A brain disorder that produces movement difficulties, most commonly among the elderly.

Pathology. The branch of medicine focusing on the laboratory-based study of disease in cells and tissues, as opposed to clinical examination of symptoms.

Pediatric. Pertaining to children.

Periodontics. The branch of dentistry focusing on the study and treatment of diseases of the bones, connective tissues, and gums surrounding and supporting the teeth.

Physiotherapy or physical therapy. The treatment or management of physical disability, malfunction, or pain by exercise, massage, hydrotherapy, and other techniques without the use of drugs, surgery, or radiation.

Plastic surgery. The branch of medicine focusing on corrective operations to the face, head, and body to restore function and (sometimes) to improve appearance (also called **cosmetic surgery**).

Polio (poliomyelitis). A paralyzing disease caused by a virus and characterized by inflammation of the motor neurons of the brainstem and spinal cord.

Positron emission tomography (PET). Also known as PET imaging or PET scanning. A diagnostic tool that captures images of the interior of the body by detecting positrons or tiny particles from radioactive material. Used to detect cancer and determine heart function; used most recently as an early clue to Alzheimer's disease. May be used in conjunction with **computed tomography (CT).**

Prosthodontics. The branch of dentistry focusing on replacing missing teeth and other oral structures with artificial devices.

Psychiatry. The branch of medicine that studies and treats mental disorders.

Radiofrequency ablation (RFA). The use of electrodes to generate heat and destroy abnormal tissue.

Radiology. The branch of medicine focusing on capturing and interpreting images, such as x-rays, CT scans, and MRI scans.

Radiosurgery. The use of ionizing radiation, either from an external source (such as an x-ray machine) or an implant, to destroy cancerous or diseased tissue.

Radiotherapy. Treatment of disease with radiation, especially by selective irradiation with x-rays or other ionizing radiation or by ingestion or implantation of radioisotopes.

Reconstructive surgery. The branch of surgery focusing on the repair or replacement of malformed, injured, or lost organs or tissues of the body, chiefly by the transplant of living tissues.

Rehabilitation. The process of restoring health and improving functioning.

Renal. Pertaining to the kidneys.

Rheumatology. The branch of medicine that studies and treats disorders characterized by pain and stiffness afflicting the extremities or back.

Stem cell. An unspecialized or undifferentiated cell that can become specialized to perform the functions of diverse tissues in the body.

Stent. A tube inserted into a blood vessel or duct to keep it open. Stents are sometimes inserted into narrowed coronary arteries to help keep them open after balloon angioplasty.

Tertiary-care. Providing care of a highly specialized nature.

Testicular epididymal sperm aspiration (TESA). A surgical procedure to obtain sperm from within the testicular tissue.

Transplant. *Organ transplant:* the surgical insertion of an organ from a donor (living or deceased) into a patient to replace an organ that is diseased or malfunctioning; transplants are available for heart, liver, lungs, pancreas, kidney, cornea, and some other organs. *Stem cell transplant:* a procedure in which stem cells are collected from the blood of the patient (autologous) or a matched donor (allogeneic) and then reinserted into the patient to rebuild the immune system. *Bone marrow transplant (BMT):* a procedure that places healthy bone marrow from the patient (autograft) or a donor (allograft) into a patient whose bone marrow is damaged or malfunctioning.

Typhoid. An infectious, potentially fatal intestinal disease caused by bacteria and usually transmitted in food or water.

Ultrasound. The use of high-frequency sound waves in therapy or diagnostics, as in the deep-heat treatment of a joint or in the imaging of internal structures.

Urology. The branch of medicine that studies and treats urinary tract infections (UTIs) and other disorders of the urinary system.

Vascular surgery. The branch of medicine focusing on the diagnosis and surgical treatment of disorders of the blood vessels, excluding the heart, lungs, and brain.

Wellness. An area of preventive medicine that promotes health and well-being though various means, such as diet, exercise, yoga, tai chi, social support, and more.

X-rays. A form of electromagnetic radiation, similar to light but of shorter wavelength, which can penetrate solids; used for imaging solid structures inside the body.

INDEX

Hospital names and specialist groups are indexed in **bold**. Main treatment categories are indexed in *italics;* specific treatments may be found in the text.

A

accommodations
  in Ankara, 192
  hospital guesthouses, 184–185
  in Izmir, 193–194
  in Kocaeli, 191
  post-treatment, 24
  proximity to treatment, 16
  recovery lodges and spas, 185–186
  scrimping on, 16
  during treatment, 24
accreditation, 44, 46–47, 81, 198–199
Acibadem Healthcare Group, 80–87
advance deposits, 40–41
aesthetic surgery. See plastic and reconstructive surgery
airfare, 22
airport transportation, 23
air transportation, 179
alcohol use while traveling, 59
Aleg, Sirmamedov, 128
algology. See pain management
allergy treatment
  Bayindir Hospital Kavaklidere, 98–100
  Bayindir Hospital Sogutozu, 100–103
all-in-one package deals, 40
Alman Hastanesi (German Hospital), 145
alternatives to JCI, 47
Alzheimer's disease treatment
  Anadolu Medical Center, 87–93
  Ankara Guven Hospital, 94–98
Anadolu Medical Center, 87–93
anesthesiology
  MESA Hospital, 134–137
Ankara, hotels in, 192
Ankara Guven Hospital, 94–98

Ankara overview, 176
anticoagulants, 58
arbitration, 28
area codes, 181
arthritis treatment. See rheumatology
assisted reproduction. See infertility treatment; IVF (in vitro fertilization); reproductive medicine
audiology
  International Hospital, 117–122
  Istanbul Memorial Hospital, 123–128
  Yeditepe University Hospital, 137–144
Australian Council of Healthcare Standards, 47

B

Bahattin, Adam, 198
banks and banking, 14, 180
bariatric surgery
  Anadolu Medical Center, 87–93
  Bayindir HealthCare Group, 98–103
  Bayindir Hospital Kavaklidere, 98–100
  Bayindir Hospital Sogutozu, 100–103
Beauty from Afar (Schult), 200
befriending the staff, 16–17
Bellroth, Natasha, 26–27
big surgeries, 44
birth control pills, 58
Blachman, Nancy, 201
blood clots in veins (DVT), 58–59
bone marrow transplantation
  in Turkey, 73–74
  Acibadem Healthcare Group, 80–87
  Anadolu Medical Center, 87–93
  Yeditepe University Hospital, 137–144
booking early, 43
Bookman, Karla R., 200
Bookman, Milica Z., 200
bottled water, 15
breast disease treatment
  Acibadem Healthcare Group, 80–87
  Yeditepe University Hospital, 137–144
BridgeHealth International, 151–152
budgeting, 21–35. *See also costs*
  airfare, 22
  Budget Planner form, 30–33
  companions, 23

ABOUT THE AUTHOR

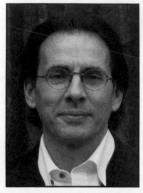

As president of Healthy Travel Media and author of *Patients Beyond Borders*, **Josef Woodman** has spent more than three years touring more than 140 medical facilities in 22 countries, researching contemporary medical tourism. As cofounder of MyDailyHealth and Ventana Communications, Woodman's pioneering background in health, wellness, and Web technology has allowed him to compile a wealth of information about global health travel, telemedicine, and new developments in consumer and institutional medical care. A noted consumer advocate for the globalization of healthcare, Woodman has lectured at Harvard Medical School and the UCLA School of Public Health, and has hosted more than a dozen seminars and workshops around the world on the topics of medical tourism and health travel.